DISEASES OF AQUARIUM FISHES

Robert Goldstein, Ph.D.
Biology Department, Emory University
Atlanta, Georgia

Distributed in the U.S.A. by T.F.H. Publications, Inc., 211 West Sylvania Avenue, P.O. Box 27, Neptune City, N.J. 07753; in England by T.F.H. (Gt. Britain) Ltd., 13 Nutley Lane, Reigate, Surrey; in Canada to the book store and library trade by Clarke, Irwin & Company, Clarwin House, 791 St. Clair Avenue West, Toronto 10, Ontario; in Canada to the pet trade by Rolf C. Hagen Ltd., 3225 Sartelon Street, Montreal 382, Quebec; in Southeast Asia by Y.W. Ong, 9 Lorong 36 Geylang, Singapore 14; in Australia and the south Pacific by Pet Imports Pty. Ltd., P.O. Box 149, Brookvale 2100, N.S.W., Australia. Published by T.F.H. Publications, Inc. Ltd., The British Crown Colony of Hong Kong.

ISBN 0-87666-041-3

CONTENTS

PREFACE

I have long felt that a book on diseases of aquarium fishes was needed and that it should combine simplicity of language with both a balanced view of the parasites most likely to be encountered and a simplified discussion of treatments. Not all flukes are skin or gill parasites, nor are they all *Gyrodactylus* or *Dactylogyrus*. Not all parasites do significant damage to fishes, and not all of them should be worried about or treated. Parasites have a place in this world; they are specialized symbionts. And many of them are far more interesting than their hosts. This book is an attempt to show them to you as I see them. Their world is generally unknown to aquarists, but it is an exciting world nevertheless.

ROBERT J. GOLDSTEIN
August, 1970

DISEASES OF AQUARIUM FISHES

1. PARASITOLOGY IN THE AQUARIUM

The parasites of aquarium fishes are not as well-known as most of us like to think. This is due to two main reasons. First, books on fish diseases emphasize the diseases of game and pond fishes and the data are drawn from experiences with American, European, and Russian pond and lake fishes of economic importance. These fishes are hosts to a number of disease agents not usually encountered in the aquarium. However, when added to what is known of aquarium fish diseases, the reader is essentially overwhelmed with names of parasites and conditions. So, the first problem is that there is too much irrelevant information. Second, and perhaps more important, is that aquarists have failed to identify and preserve those parasites which affect their fishes. This is due to the lack of a central depository for fish parasites which all aquarists ought to establish, and the unwillingness of aquarists to purchase and use a microscope.

Professional biologists in this country usually deposit specimens of the animals they work with in the Smithsonian Institution in Washington, D.C., or in the worm collection at Bethesda, Maryland. But certain conditions are attached to deposition, such as identification, origin, etc., of the specimens. Aquarists wishing to deposit specimens in a central location should send them to the proper location as directed by local fish and game authorities. A descriptive letter should accompany the specimens. Preserved fishes should be wrapped in a rag soaked in preservative and placed in a plastic bag for mailing. Do not send jars of fluid through the mails.

Diseased fishes should be placed in rubbing alcohol, or 1 part commercial formaldehyde to approximately 9 parts of tap water. If the fish is over 2 inches, its belly should be slit with a razor blade. Only living fishes should be preserved. Those that have been dead for several hours are useless unless quickly frozen and subsequently placed in preservative. Emory University is the

5

depository for the American Killifish Association and American Cichlid Association fish collections, where unusual or rare fishes are sent rather than discarded, and are thereby available for scientific taxonomic studies.

A microscope is the one item all aquarists can afford and almost none have. The aquarist should be made to understand that whereas a good research microscope that a biologist uses may cost a thousand dollars, all the aquarist needs is one that costs less than ten dollars! These children's microscopes are available at toy and hobby shops, and are usually part of kits containing many things the aquarist doesn't need. But the scope itself is important, and if one needs to buy the whole kit to get it, then that is what must be done! Usually, the eyepiece lens has a power of 10 magnification (10X), and the nosepiece contains two or three lenses (objectives) of 5X, 10X, 45X, or even 90X. It is the 10X objective lens that the aquarist most often needs. With this lens in the line of sight, the magnification is computed as the eyepiece magnification times the objective magnification, or 10X times 10X equals 100 magnification. All kits contain a booklet explaining the proper use of the microscope, and they are too simple to spend time explaining here. For the ten dollars or so, the aquarist will be able to see a whole new dimension of life, and get far more out of this most fascinating of hobbies. For example, one can see living ich and living velvet, as well as flukes, and one can observe the rapid development of the fish egg. And all for the cost of a vibrator air pump (how many do you have lying around the fish room?). After observing live aquatic creatures, one can stain them for coloration using methylene blue (washable blue ink), acriflavine, or malachite green. Or all sorts of colored inks from your stationery store!

It is difficult to handle tiny specimens for rolling around while observing them under the microscope. You should have probes and forceps. *Forceps* is the scientist's jargon for *tweezers*. That is no problem to acquire. You can make thin probes by inserting various sized needles in the eraser ends of pencils. A fine toothpick makes a dandy coarse probe.

Finally, you'll want to have small jars and formalin around for preserving your special fishes. Formalin can be acquired at your drug store or at any scientific supply house. Check the yellow pages for SCIENTIFIC or SURGICAL SUPPLY HOUSES.

And always keep formalin in your fish room medicine cabinet. It is not necessary to go to these supply houses for the various drugs used to treat most parasite infections, if you will only read the labels on the medicines at your local pet shop. Too many aquarists read the brand names rather than the ingredients, and end up with duplication rather than diversity of medications. And forget about cure-alls combining many ingredients. Use your head, not your shotgun. The drugs to look for among the ingredients are copper, acriflavine, malachite green, methylene blue, and silver salts. Let's ignore antibiotics for the present.

Finally, you should have a little table space in your fish room, with a chair and a bright lamp. Here is where you are going to use your microscope and your head. And remember, you cannot use your head effectively unless you take advantage of the written word. Your library should be adjacent to your desk, and it should be organized.

2. WHAT IS PARASITOLOGY?

Any intimate association of two species may be termed *symbiosis*. Literally, it means *living together*. Parasitism is one form of symbiosis, in which one of the organisms derives benefit at the other's expense. The parasite may be so well adapted to its host that it gets all it needs and has practically no effect on the host. This is a "smart" parasite! For if it should severely hurt or kill the host, it too will die. The more efficient the parasite, the less it harms its host. And such forms of parasitism are found widely in nature, having evolved over the milleniums. But suppose the parasite finds itself in or on an *unnatural host*. Obviously, the relationship will not be as stable as a natural one and the host is liable to be hostile to or kill the parasite, or vice-versa.

We cannot fault the parasite if it is plucked out of its natural habitat and plunked down in an aquarium of exotic fishes. The parasite is just doing its thing by infecting whatever is available and infectable. But in the unnatural environment of the aquarium one of two things usually results. Either the parasite cannot make it and is killed, or, its offensive capabilities are far and away too much for the fishes and they are rapidly decimated by a runaway parasite population. If unchecked, all the fish often die, and with them die the parasite's offspring. Nobody wins. Furthermore, if

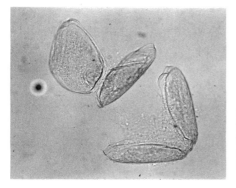

Glochidia, larval forms of freshwater mussels, which attach to fishes temporarily and can be dangerous if numerously invading gills. Goldstein photo.

the parasite has a two or three-host requirement to complete its life cycle, its chances for completion of this cycle, under aquarium conditions, are almost nil. It is doomed to failure, but it may damage or destroy some fishes along the way.

Thus, the delicate balance between the parasite and its environment (including the hosts) is very difficult to produce in artificial home aquaria, and to introduce a stage of a parasite that will next infect fishes only results in fish damage and parasite death. The study of the relationship of a species with its environment is called *ecology*. It may apply to parasites or fishes equally. The environment itself, with all its physical, biological, and chemical dynamic changes and balances, is called the *ecosystem*. The place where you find a particular species in nature is called its *habitat*. The species' place in the ecosystem (or in the *functioning* of the

Eggs of the European bitterling, *Rhodeus*, are incubated within the mantle of an adult mussel. Perkins photo.

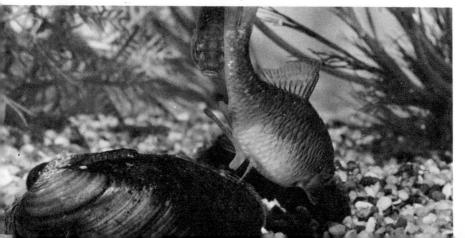

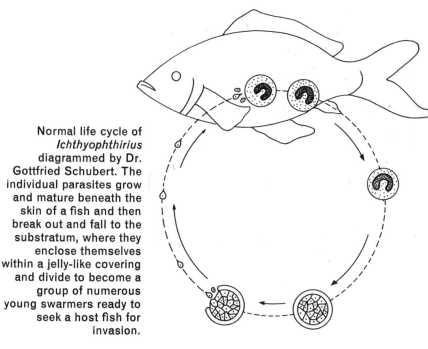

Normal life cycle of *Ichthyophthirius* diagrammed by Dr. Gottfried Schubert. The individual parasites grow and mature beneath the skin of a fish and then break out and fall to the substratum, where they enclose themselves within a jelly-like covering and divide to become a group of numerous young swarmers ready to seek a host fish for invasion.

region) is called the *ecological niche*, or just plain *niche*. It is not a place, but a function. For an example of the relationship between a parasite and all its hosts, see Goldstein (1965). Parasitology may be broadly defined as the ecology of parasites, although there are many more specific studies of parasites that are usually not considered to be ecological in nature, such as metabolism and anatomy.

3. THE ROLE OF THE NOTEBOOK

Every serious aquarist keeps a notebook in which he records data on breeding, sources of his stock, etc. Notes on diseases should also be recorded. For example, suppose your fish are infested with an epidemic of a disease. You are unable to determine which disease it is, and try all kinds of treatments (one at a time) frantically searching for a cure. Even if you *don't* find the cure, at least you have recourse to this information years later should the same thing happen. You can check your notes for a description of the symptoms, and for what did or didn't work. This will save you much irritation later, perhaps many more times than once!

4. THE CLASSIFICATION OF LIFE

As this is not a biology textbook, but one designed for serious aquarists, I shall only include categories of interest to the aquarist.

Broadly, we can consider life divided into animals, plants, and protists. Within the protists, we include bacteria (usually visible at 900X magnification), fungi (a few kinds of interest to aquarists), and viruses (not important to aquarists, generally, and sub-microscopic). The most important fish diseases, for our purposes, are either caused by bacteria or by animal parasites.

Among the animal parasites we have protozoans, such as ich, itch, and a number of things we'll cover one at a time. We also have worms, lice, and certain other interesting living things. All of these things can be seen with the naked eye and studied with a microscope or magnifying glass. Other protozoans are very small and are often internal parasites.

Among the plants, we have simple algae called dinoflagellates. A couple of species are important, and these are in the genus *Oodinium*, causing rust or velvet disease.

One fungus may be important in disease, and this is *Ichthyophonus*. It is an internal disease-producing organism. Other fungi,

Magnification of portion of a water drop; swarming infusorians are typical of abundance of life in most water environments. General Biological Supply House (Chicago) photo.

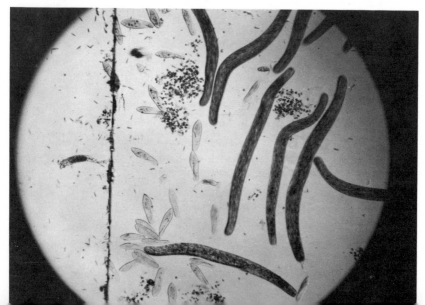

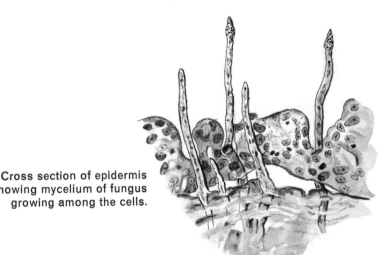

Cross section of epidermis showing mycelium of fungus growing among the cells.

such as *Saprolegnia* and *Achyla*, attack fish eggs, and sometimes an open sore of dead tissue on a living fish. The disease called "fungus" on most fish is usually a filamentous form of bacterium, and easily treated.

The bacteria are a difficult group for aquarists to diagnose. To identify bacteria, they must be studied alive in the laboratory, and preserved fish are almost worthless for making any identifications. Some bacteria are easily diagnosed by the nature of the disease (such as "fungus"), but others can cause all sorts of symptoms and diagnosis is generally not worth attempting. To determine whether a surface disease is caused by protozoans or bacteria, make a smear of the fish's surface onto a *glass slide*. (Slides are included with microscope kits, and extra ones may be purchased from the factory, or from any college bookstore.) Place a drop of water on the smear, cover with a *coverglass* (also called a coverslip: a thin glass), and observe under 100X. Most protozoans, if present, are easily seen. By cutting down the light, you will have better resolution of the unstained preparation. If nothing is seen after a 10 minute search, remove the coverglass and allow the smear to air dry naturally, without any blowing or heating. Next, pass the dry slide twice through a flame quickly, specimen side up. Stain the heat-fixed slide with methylene blue (20 minutes) or steaming hot malachite green (5 minutes) or anything else you may have available. Wash off the excess stain under a cold tap and blot dry. Observe under 900X, without a coverglass. If you have trouble seeing anything, add a drop of mineral oil to the surface of the specimen and sink the 90X objective lens into it. Now focus upward slowly until you can see something. Use maximum light. A positive bacterial diagnosis requires that the bacteria are all over the smear in enormous numbers, not merely scattered here and there. Of course, even if bacteria are found it doesn't prove that they caused the disease. But if only one kind of bacteria are present in these enormous numbers, and they are not found on smears of normal fish, you can assume that they are having a debilitating effect on the fish, whether they are primary causes of disease or not.

You can vary your staining procedures by washing with alcohol, or alcohol to which a small amount of vinegar has been added. There are many specific procedures for specific bacteria, but aquarists cannot be expected to go through such procedures and what I have outlined is perhaps sufficient. The aquarist can use his library and his head from this point onward. Unstained smears may be mailed to a parasitologist for special staining, and a covering letter explaining the symptoms in the fish should also be sent. Alternatively, the aquarist can seek out the bacteriologist, microbiologist, or parasitologist at the local university. But consider the man's time by keeping your visits few, far between, and brief; phone for an appointment before going.

The names of organisms deserve some comment. In general, all living things, except viruses, have a genus name and a specific epithet. Combined, this is the scientific name of the species, and is usually written in italics. The first letter of the genus is capitalized, but that is the only capitalized part of the entire species name. Even if the specific epithet is named after a man, it is set in lower case, e.g., *Hyphessobrycon innesi* and *Cheirodon axelrodi*. In general, an -*i* ending indicates that the critter was named after a modern man (sometimes another critter), and an -*ensis* ending is named after a place, e.g., *Cichlasoma cubensis*. A list of meanings of parts of scientific names was published in JAKA*, vol. 4, no. 3, and vol. 5, no. 1. Parasitic forms are frequently named after their hosts, e.g., *Oodinium cyprinodontum*, and *Plistophora hyphessobryconis*.

* Journal of the American Killifish Association.

A species is a member of a genus. A genus is a member of a family. A family is a member of an Order. And so on, through Class and Phylum and finally Kingdom. Biologists try to group organisms in ways that reflect their evolution. This is not always possible, and one must allow for intuition, logic, error, bias and occasionally some intended inaccuracy for the sake of convenience.

5. NON-INFECTIOUS DISEASES OF FISHES

There are a number of conditions that cause adverse effects on aquarium fishes but which are caused by other than living agents. Included here are certain types of tumors or "growths," poisoning, developmental anomalies, fright behavior and dietary degenerative diseases.

Tumors: A tumor is any abnormal multiplication of cells in the body. It usually is localized, often restricted to one tissue type, and may also be accompanied by cellular enlargement (*hypertrophy*), although cellular multiplication (*hyperplasia*) is sufficient to define the term. There is mounting evidence from studies on common laboratory animals that at least some types of tumors are caused by viruses. In general, however, we do not know the cause. Tumors are named in accordance with the types of tissues affected. For example, myomas (*myo*-muscle) are muscle tumors; lipomas (*lipo*-fat) are fatty tumors, etc. Thus, an erythrophoroma is a tumor of erythrophores, the cells containing red pigment in some fishes. We generally think of tumors as spontaneous, but in some cases we find an unusually high percentage of fishes developing them. In this type of situation one should suspect an infective

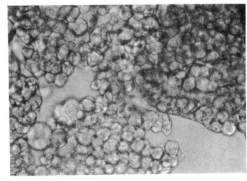

Lipoma (fatty tumor) in a serpae tetra. Goldstein photo.

13

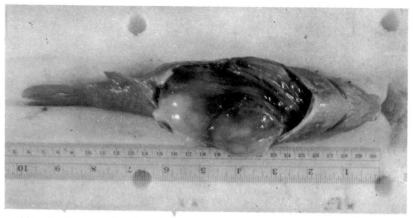
Massive tumors developed in body of a goldfish. Herman photo.

agent, a dietary deficiency or vitamin excess. Such fishes should be destroyed only if the tumor appears to be causing the fish extreme discomfort.

Poisoning: Fishes may be poisoned by direct water contamination or by the water absorbing toxic gas from the atmosphere. Frequent causes of poisoning are chlorine and chloramine. Thus, tap water should be aged (chlorine) or treated (chloramine) with sodium thiosulphate or any good chlorine or fluorine neutralizer. Three drops per gallon of a 65% solution is the recommended dechlorination concentration.

Other causes of poisoning are zinc (from washtubs or chipped refrigerator liners), paint fumes (but not from latex base paints), overdoses of malachite green, overdoses of formalin and overdoses of copper. Aquarists are quite familiar with these things. An overlooked type of poisoning of the environment is the buildup of nitrogenous wastes due to the failure of the aquarist to change a portion of the water at frequent intervals. Fishes excrete and egest nitrogenous waste products from the anus (urea) and the gills (ammonia). Some of this is converted to nitrites and nitrates by bacteria, and some of these nitrates are taken up by plants for their own protein synthesis. But aquaria are generally far more crowded than fishes are in nature, and the need for water changes cannot be overemphasized. Failure to change a third to half the water twice a month may result in optically clear, yet biologically filthy, water which can weaken the fishes, making them susceptible to ordinarily innocuous bacterial agents, or more susceptible to invasive pathogens. There is also evidence to suggest that fishes secrete substances which retard their own growth. Thus, plenty of room and very frequent water changes are most important for growing fry.

Developmental anomalies: The developmental anomaly is manifested by a fish born different. Often this is due to some biological insult it suffered during development, but I shall also include in this heading those anomalies caused by a genetic mutation. The best known example of the latter is the albino fish. This mutation causes one of the many chemical oxidative steps on the pathway to black pigment (melanin) formation to miss its

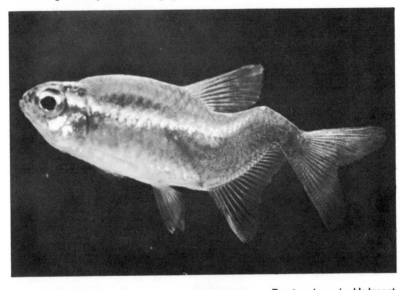

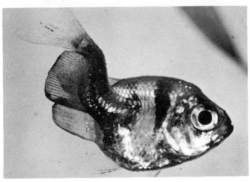

Bent spines in Helmert photo above, and in the Timmerman photo of *Gymnocorymbus ternetzi*.

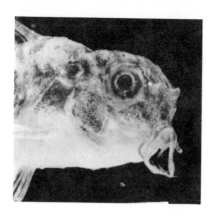

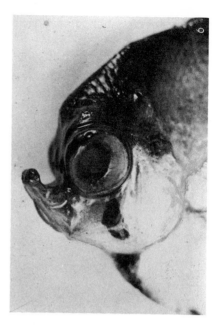

Congenitally deformed jaws.
Helmert photos.

cue, be inadequate, or be missing altogether. Since this biological mistake can occur in any of several steps, it is possible to get normally pigmented fish by crossing albinos of different strains of a species.

Another type of anomaly is the high fin, and this is also genetic. Still other examples are the different color strains of angel fishes and livebearers. All these genetic anomalies have been enjoyed and played with by aquarists. Indeed, whether something is genetic or merely a result of developmental insult can only be tested by trying to fix the anomaly in breeding.

Non-genetic anomalies include belly-sliders in killifish and mouthbrooders (dysfunction of the swim bladder), missing eyes, fins, opercula, bent spines (lordosis and kyphosis), and misshapen jaws. Aquarists are wont to blame many of these things on "in-breeding, resulting in weakening of the stock." This is nonsense. If anything, then inbreeding should select for more robust and tank-adapted fishes, and not the other way around. This erroneous thinking probably can be traced back to the general revulsion against incest and our schooling regarding the hemophilia of a line of European royalty. It is also due to a total misunderstanding of the concept of hybrid vigor. Let it suffice that these various

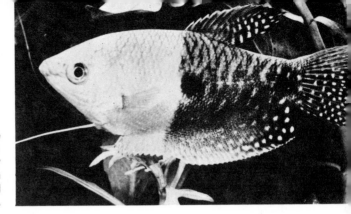

Darkening of the skin is often caused by nervous system damages. Zukal Photo.

fish anomalies are not inherited, although there is a possibility that susceptibility to environmental insult may be a characteristic of the strain or the species.

The various types of environmental damage may be caused by high temperature, handling of the eggs (by the parent fish or the aquarist), prematurity in hatching, or chemical imbalances in the water (which includes everything from direct poisoning to overdoses of malachite green or antibiotics to the wrong pH).

Dietary degenerative disease: A poorly balanced diet may result in the buildup of fatty tissue making the fish appear bloated. This may be due to liver malfunction. The liver is a key organ, and if infected or if the diet is missing elements or being overdosed with vitamins or poisons (the liver is also the principal detoxifying organ of the body), it may cause the body to either lose weight or gain fat. A fat fish can still be dying of malnutrition. At this

Tailless condition of these fish is a congenital defect. Zukal photo.

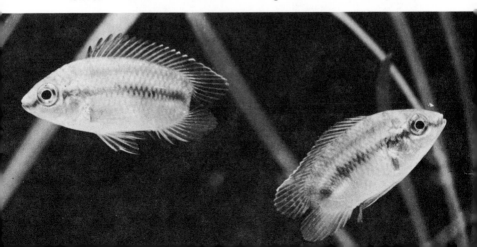

time one should also observe whether the fish is eating. If not, it should also be examined for intestinal blockage, especially if you feed raw fish, beef heart or liver. Sometimes the heavy connective tissues in the food jam the intestine and the fish slowly starves while its tissues secrete great volumes of water (edema). Suspected fishes should be treated by placing a small drop of mineral or vegetable oil in the mouth with an eyedropper. This treatment sometimes is a sufficient laxative and is especially easy to perform with catfishes (because of their large mouths), the most common victims of gut blockage.

Fright behavior: On occasion, aquarists and dealers are befuddled by a tankful of fishes (usually of the same species) that go wild, dashing about the tank, and out of it, and often bumping the walls and even killing themselves. One explanation is available now, but it doesn't answer all cases. In the skin of the fish are two types of important cells; the slime cells which are open to the

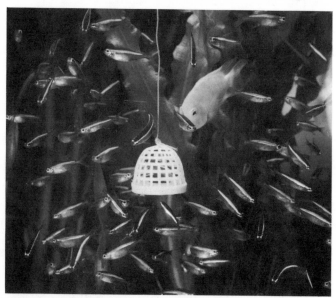

Nutritional freeze-dried foods are favored by many aquarists.

surface by pores and produce the slimy protective coating; and the club cells which are not open to the surface. When a fish is wounded, some of these club cells are exposed to the water and empty their contents. Fish of the same or related species can smell this substance and it causes them to flee wildly. Assumedly, this is an adaptation which protects fish of the same species from a predator in dark waters. But these club cells and *fright substance* which they release have been found in only certain major groups of fishes. And this does not explain why the same thing can happen in a tank where a fish has apparently not been wounded (by either a predator or by one of its own kind). Fright substances are rather specific. The more closely related two species, the more likely that one will be frightened by injury to the other. There are no accepted methods for dealing with this phenomenon, other than uncrowding the fish and making a water change.

6. VIRUS DISEASES

A virus is quite different from any other form of life. It carries on no metabolic activities of its own. Its parasitism has advanced so far that all it needs to do is invade a host cell and "tell" the cell what to do. Upon invasion, the cell stops working for itself and begins to work for the virus. From then on, the sole fucntion of the cell is to produce more virus.

A virus consists of next to nothing. It has a core of genetic material, surrounded by a protective sheath of protein. During or after it invades the host cell, the protein coat is shed, and the viral genetic material directs the host cell's activity. The host cell proceeds to make new viral genetic material and new viral protein. Eventually these are put together to form many new virus particles and the particles leave the cell. The cell may now persist with its machinery in disarray, or it may die. The whole cycle of invasion, production, and release may take less than an hour, or it may take years. The number of kinds of viruses is staggering and they may infect higher animals, plants, bacteria, and lower animals (invertebrates); this last category is the most recent to be discovered.

A small number of fish viruses are known, almost all of them from game fishes. As you might expect, parasites are where you look for them, and people look at those animals for which there are research funds. Is it any wonder then, that there is only one virus documented from an aquarium fish? Even this one, ironically, was first discovered and has been most studied in game fishes.

The virus is called Lymphocystis Virus. (Note that names of viruses are not arranged as genus and species, and are not italicized.

Viruses are subject to neither the Laws of Zoological nor Botanical Nomenclature. And they are not bacteria either, and so even that poor set of rules does not apply.) Lymphocystis Virus has been known for half a century, and was discovered due to its strange effect on the host cell. When the cell is invaded, it enlarges enormously, up to 100,000 times in volume. Ken Wolf of the Eastern Fish Diseases Laboratory has described the infection sites as resembling a spattering of farina, and the larger masses having a raspberry texture. These lesions are the result of groups of infected cells, each cell attaining a size of perhaps a millimeter (one twenty-fifth of an inch).

The virus itself is incredibly small, although large as viruses go! Its size is given as 300 mμ, which is 0.3μ. One μ (pronounced *micron*) is equal to one thousandth of a millimeter. And so the virus particle is three ten-thousandths of a millimeter!

Lymphocystis Virus occurs naturally in centrarchid fishes (basses, perch, sunfish) in fresh waters. It can now be propagated in laboratory reared centrarchid tissue cells, where fish cells are grown under special conditions and propagated.

The enlarged cells resulting from Lymphocystis invasion have been called tumor cells, but the tumors are localized and generally do not cause death.

The virus has been found naturally in Guatemala in the cichlid fish, *Cichlasoma synspilum*. In some ways the virus-induced cellular changes differ in this one cichlid from previous reports in centrarchids. In any case, it is clear that if the virus can grow in one cichlid, it probably can grow in others. Aquarists should watch for small growths on the surfaces of their cichlids (and other fishes), and contact the editors of the hobby magazines if they wish to donate the fish to a researcher.

There is no cure for the virus, short of cutting out the infected tissue. But other cells on the fish may also carry the virus, and they may not yet be visible (or internal cells may be infected). One should keep in mind that viruses, in general, cannot be treated with drugs. More important, this particular virus is not expected to cause death or even great debilitation in your fish. As with many other parasites, then, the best approach is to leave it alone.

There are several other virus diseases of fishes, but these have no relation to aquarium fishes and will not be discussed here.

7. BACTERIAL DISEASES OF FISHES

There are many kinds of bacteria that cause disease in fishes. The disease may be *primary* (the bacterium is a known, very invasive pathogen), or *secondary* (bacteria that grow where the fish has already been damaged). Some bacteria are only occasional disease producers, others produce disease under conditions which stress the fish, and still others produce diseases in some fishes but not in others. One of the difficulties in identifying bacterial diseases is that a single *agent* may cause different symptoms in different fish or water conditions. In a community tank some fish may die with no apparent marks or lesions, while others continue to live for a while, but with whitish ulcerations or patches on the body. If these fishes had been in separate aquaria, the aquarist would be led to believe that different diseases were at work.

Another problem in diagnosis of a disease stems from the nature of bacterial taxonomy itself. Bacteria are classified only partly on their shape (round: *coccus*, rod-like: *bacillary*, and twisted or curved: *spirillum*). They are also classed on whether they have *flagella* (little whip-like extensions enabling them to swim), and if so, then where they are located (at the end of the cell: *polar*; or all around the cell: *peritrichous*).

Most important, they are classified on the cell's chemical properties and metabolic activities. This means that bacteria must be studied alive for an accurate diagnosis. This involves testing them to see if they can use certain sugars for growth, whether they break down proteins, fats, or other odd types of molecules, and whether they produce certain metabolic waste products (and if so, in what concentrations). Thus, a pickled or even freshly dead fish is often insufficient for doing the necessary laboratory work leading to a correct identification. And this laboratory work is considerable. Some animal parasites are distinct in enough anatomical properties for an experienced parasitologist to make a rapid identification. But the same is almost never true with bacteria; thus, they are difficult to identify.

With all these problems, what can the aquarist do? Fortunately, bacteria fall into three general categories based on staining reactions. A small percentage of bacteria are positive for the *acid-fast stain*. These bacteria are generally slow growers, distantly related to human tuberculosis and leprosy, but of no danger in

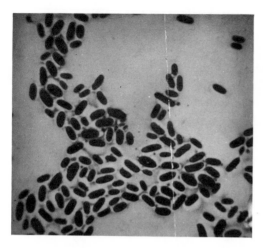

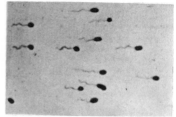

*Bacterium
lepidorthosae*, C. van
Duijn, Jr. photo; (right)
Pseudomonas punctata,
after Schäperclaus.

any real sense to aquarists. They most often are found in external sores or internal lesions in very old fishes. These acid-fast bacteria are all in the genus *Mycobacterium*. Because they grow so slowly, it is difficult to use antibiotics to interfere with their cellular machinery. Thus, the best treatment for such infections is disposal of the few infected and old specimens. Generally, these bacteria may be found in old annual killifishes, and probably contribute to speeding up the very rapid aging process. One does not ordinarily get epidemics of such a disease, and we need not concern ourselves any longer with this very small group.

The other two groups are separated on the basis of another laboratory staining reaction, developed by Christian Gram. This reaction tells us something of the nature of the cellular wall surrounding the bacterium. The staining procedure is easy to perform, rapid, but requires that the bacteria are taken from a pure culture less than 24 hours old. Thus, aquarists cannot be expected to perform this test. Bacteria are either Gram positive or Gram negative by this staining reaction. This has important implications for treatment, as most antibiotics on the market are selective for one or the other class of bacteria.

Gram-Positive Bacteria: This category is of practically no concern to aquarists. If the bacterial cells are numerous, short rods, and with a tendency to occur in pairs, and if you find them in the kidneys (and perhaps other viscera), the bacteria are probably in the genus *Corynebacterium*. These are not known from

Acid-fast bacterium (Mycobacterium sp., red-stained here), rod-like bacteria tending to occur in packets, from skin lesion of a Venezuelan longfin, *Pterolebias longipinnis*. Goldstein photo.

fishes of aquarium interest. If the cells are acid-fast, long, thin, and few in number, you probably have one of the species of *Mycobacterium*. The fish should be considered a lost cause anyway; the tank need not be treated other than giving it a good siphoning and partial water change.

Gram-Negative Bacteria: One well known form is called *Chondrococcus columnaris* and is the agent causing *columnaris* or *cotton wool disease*. It is world-wide in distribution, and may occur on any kind of fish. The sores are manifested as gray or whitish spots on the body with a tendency to rapidly spread. Generally, many fish show the symptoms at once, indicating rapid spread and high contagion. The bacteria are very long and slender, easily seen under the microscope, and seem to bend or creep. The disease is very common in aquaria and rapidly fatal. The tank water should be mostly replaced with new water, the bottom siphoned, and the tank treated with an antibiotic plus methylene blue. The dye will lower the overall bacterial count in the water, which might have contributed to the fish becoming susceptible.

Other diseases are manifested as blood spots, swelling, opaque areas on the flesh, fin and tail rot, dropsy, etc. These may be caused by a number of species and even more numerous strains of *Aeromonas* and *Pseudomonas*. Some are contagious and others are not. In most cases, dirty tanks or unchanged water (with a great build-up of nitrogenous wastes) may be considered the primary insult which weakened the fish to become susceptible to the disease. Shipping fishes in crowded containers without tranquilizers may also constitute adequate insults to get the diseases started. Most of these bacteria are very short, rod-shaped cells, and may be motile (having flagella) or not motile. There is no way to make a diagnosis strictly by using a microscope.

Aeromonas punctata has been reported from barbs in India, and the closely similar genus *Paracolobactrum* has been reported from *Corydoras*, *Xiphophorus* and *Poecilia*. Information on disease-causing bacteria of tropical fishes is very sparse, frequently poorly documented, and not yet large enough to constitute a body of knowledge worthy of the title, *science*. The fault lies not with lack of effort, but with lack of interested persons.

Treatment: In all bacterial diseases, the first thing to be done is change most of the water and siphon the bottom detritus. Massive doses of methylene blue dye will cut down the overall bacterial population, but may affect some kinds of plants. One should treat the fish with antibiotics. Note that antibiotics are used only for bacterial (and some fungal) diseases, and never for protozoa! Old fish should be destroyed, as should those which are very seriously debilitated and probably beyond treatment.

In most cases, Gram-positive bacteria can be ruled out. The exception is for filament-like growths on the fish which may or may not be fungus. Swab the growth with household mercurochrome and treat the tank with *penicillin*. This antibiotic specifically interferes with the formation of cell walls of these bacteria and is the drug of choice. There are several derivatives of penicillin, so know your product.

There are many drugs which attack Gram-negative cells. We generally use *tetracycline, chloramphenicol, sulfonamides,* or *streptomycin*. Penicillin has no effect, because the cell walls of these bacteria are made differently. Most of these drugs are *analogues* of substances the bacteria need for normal growth (multiplication). They pick up these structurally similar compounds by mistake, and end up fouling up their own cellular machinery. Naturally, antibiotics must be substances which fool bacteria but not higher organisms. This is why you can use penicillin (higher animals don't have cell walls at all), but not cyanide or strychnine poisons. Use only one antibiotic when treating one disease. Follow the directions on the labels of any of the commercial preparations. Do not use streptomycin in a tank that has a colony of *Tubifex* growing

Principles of antibiotic chemotherapy: (1) *para-amino-sulfanilic acid* ("sulfanilamide") is a drug that fools bacteria into thinking they are getting (2) *para-amino-benzoic acid*, a substance they require for normal functioning. (3) *chloramphenicol* interferes with bacterial protein synthesis, but is a dangerous drug for humans, and only used in emergency situations. (4) *penicillin* occurs in several forms, where the –R– group may be varied. It interferes with bacterial cell wall synthesis. (5) *tetracylines* also occur in several forms, and inhibit protein synthesis. (6) *streptomycins* cause bacteria to mis-read their genetic instructions and make mistakes in protein synthesis.

25

on the bottom. These worms are very sensitive to the drug, will die, and their carcasses will result in more bacterial growth. This drug will also result in the build-up of aromatic organic compounds in about a week. The tank will have a sickly sweet odor. For this reason, treatment with antibiotics should be followed by an almost total water change after three days. As soon as the drug is no longer needed, get rid of it.

Antibiotics should never be used as "tonics," as they are indiscriminate in that they destroy not only pathogens, but many useful bacteria as well.

8. FUNGUS DISEASES

The study of fungi (pronounced FUN'-JYE) is called *mycology*. Today it is a neglected branch of biology, and there are too few people trained and involved in it compared with the enormous number of forms known.

Fungi are a varied group of organisms, many of them closely related to certain bacteria (such as the acid-fast bacteria), and still others hardly related to each other at all. Some cause filamentous

Saprolegnia, a fungus well known to aquarists. Helmert photo.

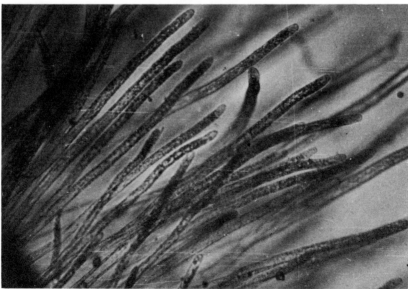

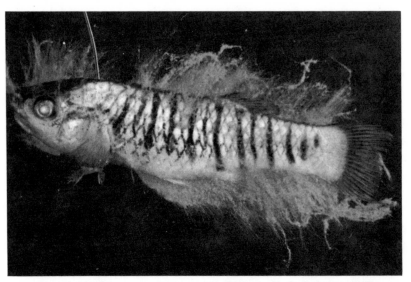

A dead fish is soon consumed by fungus. M. F. Roberts photo.

growths in or on fishes (and other animals), and others have ameboid stages and cysts. Many are hard to recognize for what they are. The fungi contain parasites with the most complex life cycles known, several agricultural pests having as many as seven required hosts in the life cycle. Examples of fungi are athlete's foot, ringworm, plant rust and plant wilt, mushrooms, toadstools, etc. The few species known from fishes reflects lack of study, not lack of parasites.

The best known fungi of aquarium fishes are species of *Achyla* and *Saprolegnia*. Normally, these fungi grow on dead fish eggs (every cichlid breeder has seen them on a large portion of eggs), but they may occur on dead and uneaten food in the aquarium. Most importantly, they sometimes invade wounds in the skin of fishes and appear as cottony or wooly growths at the site of damage. Only a small portion of the fungus is visible on the wound, most of the parasitic material growing inside the wound. Such cases of fungus at a wound should be treated by removing the fish in a net and swabbing the wound with household mercurochrome. The fish should be returned to a tank of clean water devoid of other fishes; otherwise other fishes are liable to pick at the wound and aggravate the situation. To prevent or retard the build-up of fungi on fish eggs in a breeding tank, the water should contain acriflavine dye. There are many commercial remedies available, and the aquarist should follow the directions on the label. This dye breaks down rapidly in light, and always comes in a dark bottle. If the aquarist can prepare his own from powdered dye, a dark bottle should be used for storage, and only a small quantity made at a time. The strength of the prepared solution is not very important, so long as the prepared solution is reddish, and drops placed in an aquarium rapidly assume a green color. Acriflavine preparations are actually a mixture of various flavin dyes, and I do not believe there is any great difference in effectiveness or usefulness among the available preparations.

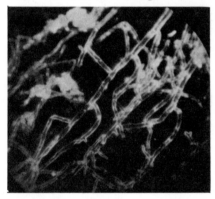

C. van Duijn, Jr. photomicrograph of fungus filaments from a fish.

There has been a lot of misinformation published about another fungus, *Ichthyophonus*. This is a genus of parasitic organisms occurring in the organs and tissues of many marine and some freshwater fishes. It is supposed to be widespread among aquarium fishes, but I have encountered it at autopsy only rarely. A word about the proper generic name. It seems that many organisms have been called *Ichthyophonus* or *Ichthyosporidium*. As a matter of fact, it turns out that some of these cases dealt with true fungus infection, and others dealt with an unusual type of protozoan infection. With ordinary staining procedures, these two diseases are difficult to tell apart. However, with the periodic acid/Schiff stain (referred to in the literature as PAS), the protozoan structure can be seen. At present, biologists are restricting the name *Ichthyophonus* for the fungus species, and *Ichthyosporidium* for the protozoan species. The older literature, you must understand, con-

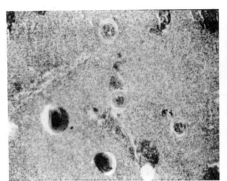
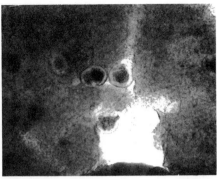
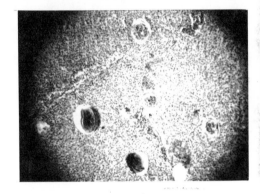

Unidentified fungus in
liver of a discusfish.
Goldstein photos.

fuses the two as caused by the same kind of organism. This has
great bearing on choosing a treatment.

The treatment for *Ichthyophonus* is somewhat involved, and a
careful diagnosis of the disease should precede any medication
other than the use of formalin. (Formalin attacks many kinds of
parasites, including protozoa, and may be used first in an attempt
to correct conditions in a "sick" tank.) The fungus causes hard
whitish-yellow spots to occur in several organs, including the liver
(easiest to locate). The freshly dead fish should be removed and
examined for signs of major external injury. If this can be ruled
out as a cause of death, the fish is next slit open with a razor blade
and its liver removed and examined. Even if no spots are visible,
crush a bit of the liver between your fingers. If it feels sandy, you
can suspect this fungus. Make a smear on a glass slide and examine
under the low power of your microscope. Compare what you find
with the photos in this book. *Ichthyophonus* cysts are generally
clustered and have a thick rim and rather amorphous interior (the

interior is the ameboid *plasmodium*; the rim is the wall of the *cyst*). Don't be surprised if you find something not illustrated in this book. There are many kinds of fungi and protozoa that infect the viscera of fishes, and we only know a small part of the true story. If something new is found (or if you want verification of your diagnosis), preserve the remaining tissue in formalin (one part stock solution to 9 parts tap water) and send it to the editor of a hobby magazine for forwarding to a competent and interested biologist.

If your diagnosis is positive for *Ichthyophonus*, the first thing to be done is to rapidly remove dying fishes from the aquarium. The disease may be spread by a healthy fish feeding on the carcass of one dead of the disease, thereby ingesting the infection himself. The second thing to do is set up the hospital tank for treatment with *phenoxyethanol*. This drug is also called *phenoxethol*, but that name is not in favor today in the U.S.A. There is a stronger (more potent) preparation called *para*-chloro-phenoxyethanol, but it is difficult to come by. Ordinary phenoxyethanol works well enough for our purposes. It is available at scientific supply and drug firms, and you should consult your yellow pages for a dealer. You

Ichthyophonus hoferi in liver of a flounder. Goldstein photo.

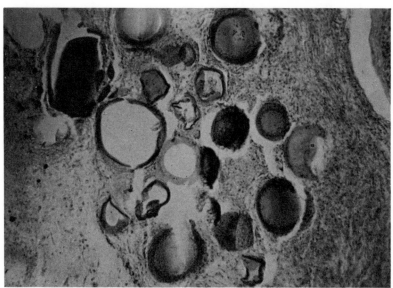

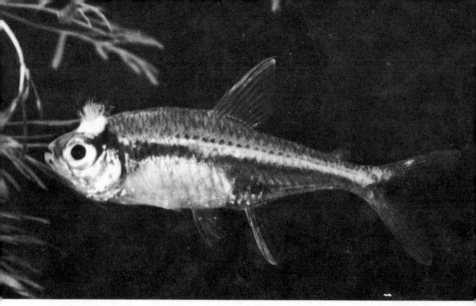

Fungus invasion of head injury of *Hyphessobrycon heterorhabdus*. Zukal photo.

will also need some glass pipettes, graduated in milliliters (*ml*'s, also called cubic centimeters or *cc*'s). A milliliter is one thousandth of a liter, and a liter is approximately a quart. The drug is a very viscous liquid, and it has a low solubility in water. You must use very hot water to get it into solution. The maximum dose is about one *ml* per gallon of water in the hospital tank. Suppose you have a ten gallon tank. Get a gallon jar or a quart jar, and fill it with very hot water from the tap. Add ten *ml* of the drug (using the pipette) to this hot water and stir until you have a clear solution (which will take plenty of stirring). Add about a third of this solution to the tank every 12 hours, or until the fish show signs of drowsiness. Once drowsiness has been achieved, stop adding the drug. It is a general anaesthetic and too much can kill the fish. Because different species have different tolerances to the drug, we use the one *ml* concentration (per gallon) as the upper limit, a limit you should not ordinarily have to attain.

There is no set of symptoms that will enable you to diagnose the disease. An autopsy is necessary. The effectiveness of the drug is still not well known, but it is all we have available. If you can get the *para*-chloro derivative of the drug, cut the dosage to a tenth of what has been described above.

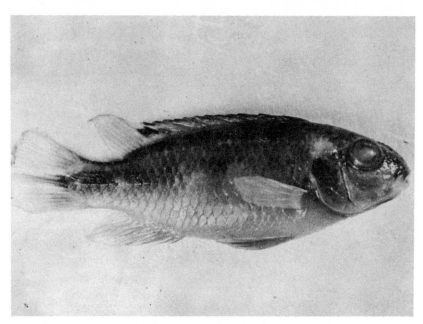

Typical appearance of fishes attacked by *Ichthyosporidium*. Helmert photos.

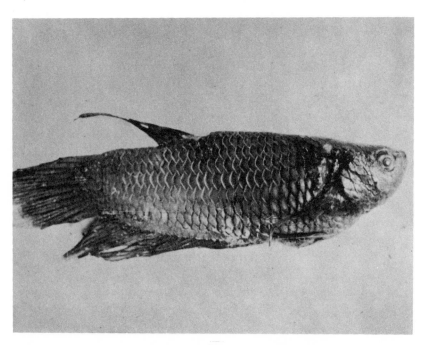

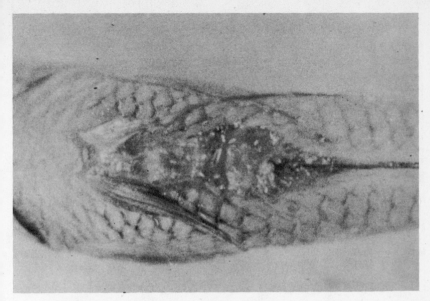
Belly growths of fish with *Ichthyophonus*. Helmert photo.

9. ALGAE

Aquarists seldom think of algae as disease producers, if they think of them at all. Actually the term *algae* is even broader than the term *fish*. There are blue-green algae, green, red, brown, and other algae, and each of these categories makes up an entire phylum of organisms. The green algae contains many organisms of biological interest, and it is from these organisms that the higher plants are though to have evolved. One group, the DINO-FLAGELLATES, is characterized by having a pair of whiplike flagella in a special arrangement, and some other criteria. Being green algae, the dinoflagellates contain a number of pigments common to the phylum, some of them involved in the conversion of light energy into chemical energy.

The genus *Oodinium* is an unusual genus of dinoflagellates, in that it contains parasites. Most species are parasitic on marine fishes, but two are of interest to the American aquarist. The first is *Oodinium limneticum*, the causative agent of *rust* or *velvet* disease. This is the only freshwater species of the genus known, and can attack almost any kind of aquarium fish. It is the only disease that can truly be called the bane of killifish fanciers, but its occurrence is far wider than generally realized. Velvet kills lots of fry.

The second species of interest is the newly discovered (1967) *Oodinium cyprinodontum*, a parasite of estuarine killifishes in the United States. There has been no work published to date on the salinity tolerance of this species, but it is well known that estuarine animals (and plants) in general tolerate considerable fluctuations in salinity, often ranging from marine water (sp. g. 1.025) to practically freshwater. As various American native killifishes become established in aquaria, this species of velvet will probably be found more frequently.

Unlike "ich," the agent of velvet attaches to the skin or gills of the fish, and only sends its little root-like rhizoids into the host. The body of the parasite remains outside where it is susceptible to various available treatments. This stage is called the *trophont* (*troph*—to eat). The trophont varies from microscopic to easily visible, but it never attains the size of the ich organism. The body

Oodinium limneticum, the golden, dust-fine parasitic agent of velvet disease, attached to skin of a *Nothobranchius* killifish. Goldstein photo.

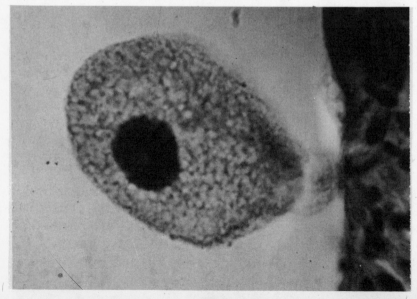

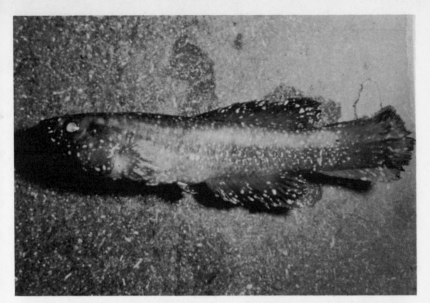

Ichthyophthirius in a golden pheasant, *Roloffia occidentalis*; spots are larger, brighter, and less numerous than in velvet. Goldstein photo.

is teardrop shaped, and the little rhizoids at the narrow end are very difficult to see even with good microscopic equipment. There is some yellowish pigment, and this becomes apparent in a heavy infection.

A light infection will go unnoticed in any aquarist's fish room, but when a fish comes down with a heavy infection (all too frequently!), the body and fins are seen to be covered with a very fine, dusty material that looks like rust. These are the thousands of *O. limneticum* trophonts. They are most easily seen by playing a very bright light on the fish.

When the trophont reaches its maximal size, it drops from the fish and encysts. During the next few days it multiplies rapidly, and a single cyst may divide to form very many (about 250) little swimming parasites. These little swimmers are called swarmers or dinospores. In *O. cyprinodontum* there may be over 2000 dinospores formed from a single cyst. As you might expect, these dinospores have the flagella characteristic of dinoflagellates. Of course, they lose them when they attach to a fish.

Velvet is a disease of dirty tanks. If fish are kept in clean water and the bottom is regularly siphoned, the disease almost never occurs. The filthy tank containing uneaten meats, soil or peat moss, excessive droppings, etc., is almost invariably associated with outbreaks. Some fishes are far more susceptible than others. This is especially true of young tetras, rasboras, and killifish, especially species of *Nothobranchius*. Velvet has been blamed on live food, dried food, frozen food, etc., but aquarists almost never blame the outbreaks on their own dirty housekeeping, and that is the only place the blame should lie.

Treatment is with copper or malachite green. Other treatments are available, but these are the best. Malachite green often kills tetras and some other fishes in dosages required to have it operate (about 1 drop per gallon of a 0.75% aqueous solution), and copper should be considered the drug of choice.

Fishes vary in the susceptibility to copper poisoning, and the chemistry of the aquarium water will determine what portion of the copper input is actually available as a disease fighter. And so there is no set dosage. But we do know that velvet and snails are both very sensitive to the drug, and this gives us a method of treatment.

If there are no snails in the tank, put some in. Begin adding copper sulfate solution until the snails begin to drop from the glass and plants. When all the snails have finally given up the ghost, you have added more than enough of the drug to wipe out the velvet. Take out the dead snails, wait 24 hours, and then replace two-thirds of the aquarium water with new water (dechlorinated).

If you wish to use malachite green, you can use the 0.75% solution as indicated above (one drop per gallon), or as a dip. If used as a dip take the fish in a net, dip it for no more than a second in the concentrated dye, dip it in a bucket of clean water for washing, and then return it to its aquarium.

The presence of *Oodinium* on the outside of the fish, rather than imbedded deep under the skin, makes it easy to cure, provided one uses high doses of drugs. Failures to effect cures can be traced to low dosages. Velvet is a deadly disease and should be treated promptly.

10. PROTOZOAN DISEASES

The protozoa constitute a very large phylum of single celled animals, many of which are parasitic in or on fishes and other animals. For the sake of convenience, we will use a simplified system of classification.

Class 1. Ciliophora   = ciliated protozoa
Class 2. Mastigophora = flagellated protozoa
Class 3. Sarcodina   = amoeboid protozoa
Class 4. Sporozoa   = all species parasitic

Examples of Ciliophora, or "ciliates," would include *Paramecium*, that most frequent constituent of infusoria cultures, and *Ichthyophthirius*, the causative agent of ich or white spot disease.

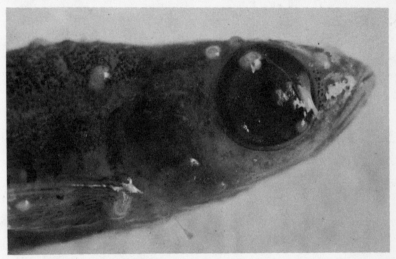

Ichthyophthiriasis patches (enlarged here). Helmert photo.

The ciliates have bands or patches of fine, hair-like, protein threads over the surface of the body, and these threads (or *cilia*) beat in a wave-like motion. In some specialized forms, such as *Trichodina*, clusters of these cilia may be modified into tooth-like grasping appendages. This is analogous to the horn of a rhinoceros, which consists of tightly woven clusters of hair.

Ichthyophthirius multifiliis is the only species of ich. It may occur on any kind of fish, anywhere in the world. The free-swimming parasite invades the skin of a fish, often when the fish has been stressed, burrows under the epithelium, and derives nourishment and grows. After it achieves a large size (and is recognized as white spots seemingly *on* rather than actually just *under* the skin), it breaks out of the skin and drops to the bottom of the aquarium. During the next two to four days (depending on temperature), the cell divides many times to produce a large number of daughter parasites. When division has been completed, the cyst breaks down and the baby ciliated parasites swim away looking for another fish to invade. It is only during this free-swimming stage that the aquarist can kill the parasite. For while it remains in its cyst on the floor of the tank, or while it resides in the skin of the fish, drugs will not harm it.

The drug of choice is malachite green (1 drop of a 0.75% aqueous solution per gallon). Formalin (4 drops of commercial pre-parations per gallon) or acriflavine (follow the directions on the bottle) are used on tetras, as these fishes do not tolerate malachite green dye.

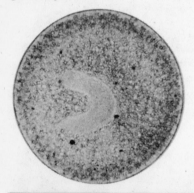

Helmert photo of *Ichthyophthirius*; (below) a cluster photographed by the author. Note horseshoe-shaped nucleus.

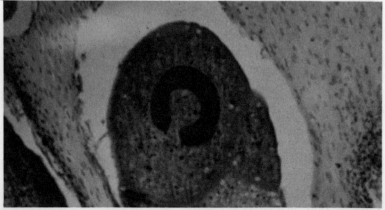

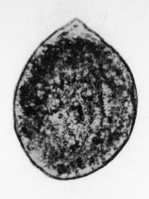

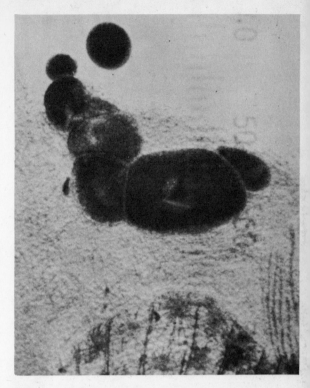

Spore of *Ichthyophthirius* and (right) tissue of infested fish showing parasites in various stages of development. Helmert photos.

Ichthyophthirius multifiliis was once said to be a possible skin invader of man, but that report has been firmly squelched by Reichenbach-Klinke.

Trichodina occurs more often in aquarium literature than it does in freshwater aquaria! It is a beautiful parasite, its cilia forming rings of *denticles*. About one hundred species of *Trichodina* have been recorded in the literature from freshwater and marine fishes. About 20 freshwater species are known from the United States, and there is some evidence that they are rather (or slightly) host-specific in nature. What happens in the aquarium is anybody's guess. However, the lack of reports of *Trichodina* on aquarium fishes (with few exceptions) would indicate either or both of two points: (1) their specificity in nature is carried over into aquaria so that native fishes do not cause aquarium epidemics of exotics; (2) they are more common than realized, because people just don't look for them. *Trichodina* (and related genera) are easily recognized under the microscope, and specimens should be saved for species identification by an expert.

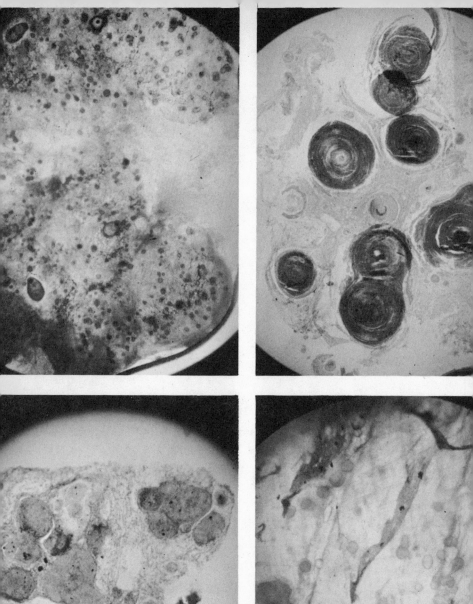

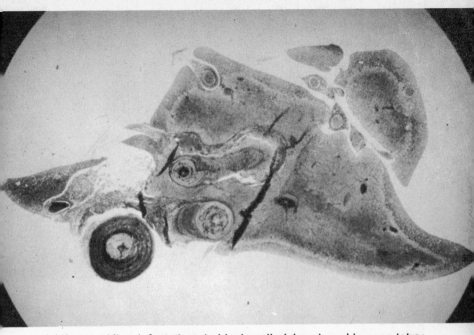

Ichthyosporidium infestations in black molly (above), and in neon tetra; (on facing page) in *Betta splendens* in upper photos and in *Hyphesso-brycon ornatus* in the lower ones. Geisler photos.

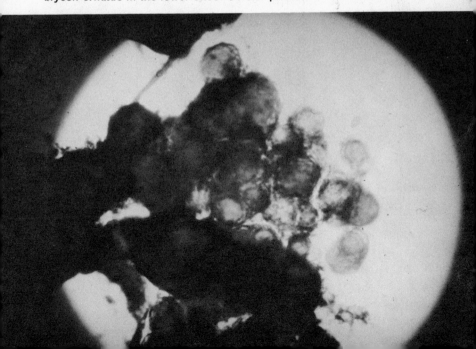

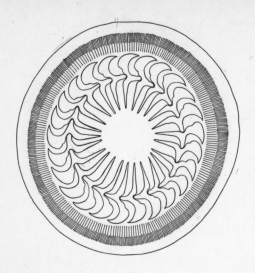

Diagrammatic
representation of
Trichodina (protozoan
ectoparasite responsible
for itching symptoms and
fin degeneration),
showing adhesive disc,
denticles, radial pins, and
border membrane.

Cryptobia salmositica, a flagellate protozoan of salmonid fishes. The large, clear cells with dark nuclei are fish blood cells; the parasites appear granular and almost as large. Goldstein photo.

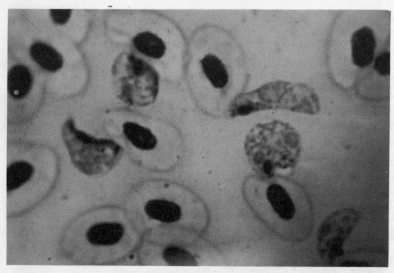

Treatment of choice is formalin, as for *Ichthyophthirius*. The parasites reside on, rather than in, the skin and are thus susceptible to the action of the drug immediately. Acriflavine is also effective, but formalin is cheaper, and may be used on any superficial protozoan infestation of fishes.

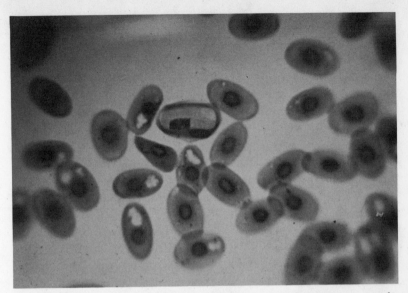

Haemoproteus, a member of the sporozoan type of protozoans and causative agent of a form of animal malaria; the parasite (with rectangular nucleus) is shown in the center of the field and occupying most of a single red cell of turtle blood. Goldstein photo.

The Class Mastigophora contains the *flagellates*. These animals have whip-like extensions resembling cilia, but there are fewer of them, they are much longer, and they do not beat in a wave-like motion. Of course, there are other differences as well. Examples of flagellates are the blood parasites of African sleeping sickness, the protozoa in the gut of termites which enable these animals to digest wood, and certain free-living forms. *Oodinium* is sometimes classified in this group of Protozoa, but we have already seen that most biologists classify it as a member of the plant kingdom, in the green algae.

There are several genera of flagellates of fishes, but the generic divisions are often unclear. Thus, *Hexamita* and *Octomitis* are very close and may even be identical. If so, then *Hexamita* is the older and valid name. *Hexamita truttae* is an intestinal parasite of various game fishes, but is also known from *Pterophyllum scalare*, *Heterandria formosa*, and *Cichlasoma severum*. Obviously, it is not host-specific at all, and could cause epidemics in aquaria. *Spironucleus elegans* has been reported from the gut of *Pterophyllum scalare*. A species of *Hexamita-Octomitis* (?) has been seen in discus fish. There are no aquarium remedies available for these intestinal parasites, although Carbarsone and Calomel are used in hatcheries. I would suggest that you seek these ingredients in some anthelminthic dog and cat foods, and use these foods for your fishes. These drugs combat intestinal amoebae in pet mammals, and sometimes occur in shotgun-approach drugged foods. Or phone your local veterinarian. Flagellates are easily diagnosed by their whiplike motion in the intestinal fluids at autopsy. Flagyl is a new drug recommended on an experimental basis.

The Class Sporozoa is no longer recognized by biologists, but we will use it for protozoa that have neither cilia, flagella, nor amoeboid forms of motility. They develop spores at some stage in the life cycle, and all species are parasitic. They divide asexually (schizogony; *schizo*-split) and sexually (sporogony). They may occur in any organ or tissue, and may or may not require a *vector* (transmitter of the disease). [Malaria of man is caused commonly by three species of sporozoa, but in that case, the mosquito is the definitive host and man serves as intermediate host and vector! (If the mosquito gets sick, it's because it drank from a contaminated person.)]

The Coccidia are a large group of sporozoans, occurring in blood and intestinal cells. One huge genus is *Eimeria*, infecting fishes, man, and farm animals, and almost anything else that is examined for them. *Eimeria aurati* occurs in goldfish, but there are other species in this and related fishes. The feces may be long, white and opaque in heavy (the only kind?) infections, and the cysts are then very abundant. The presence of this type of dropping does not indicate infection with *Eimeria*, necessarily, and microscopic examination is imperative. There is no treatment known.

Closely related to the Coccidia are the Haemosporidea, containing the genus *Babesiosoma*. These are parasites of the red blood cells, and while probably rare in aquarium fishes, ought to be easily found (if not recognized to genus).

In order to find blood parasites, the aquarist must learn to make a proper blood smear. One needs two very clean glass microscope slides. A clean drop of blood (get it any way you can!) is placed on

44

one end of one slide, and the slide rested on a table. The other slide is placed at a 45 degree angle, and slid along the first slide until it touches the drop of blood. Now the blood will spread out along the leading edge of the held (angled) slide. This slide is then pulled back, dragging the blood with it, and forming a thin film. The held slide is now discarded or cleaned and put away. The slide containing the blood film is allowed to air dry, and sent to an expert for evaluation following staining. The staining procedure is too complex for aquarists.

Babesiosoma (*Dactylosoma*) *mariae* was reported from four species of *Haplochromis* cichlids from Lake Victoria, Uganda, and subsequently from other cichlids and cyprinids from the same region. It is the only species known from aquarium fishes, or potential aquarium fishes. Other species occur in frogs, salamanders and marine fishes. A species has recently been found in a freshwater fish in the United States.

So much for Coccidea and Haemosporidea. A third group (and the most important) is the Cnidospora. The Cnidospora contains the Myxosporidea and Microspirodea. They usually form cysts in the tissues, and each cyst may contain a few to many spores, but sometimes only a single spore is formed. Classification is on the number and morphology of the spores. The Myxosporidea usually have bivalvular cysts, i.e., the appearance of "pairs," and are rather large. The Microsporidea are generally smaller, and the cysts appear single. The Myxosporidea are the larger group.

Among the Myxosporidea, *Myxosoma* invades cartilage, often of the gill arches. There are about 50 described species; about 30 from North American fishes. They are probably quite host and tissue specific, and there thus seems to be little chance of epidemics in aquaria. No treatment available, other than destruction of fishes and sterilization of aquaria. Aquarium information is lacking.

Another Myxosporidian is *Henneguya*. It may invade the fin rays, the eye, gills, or fin tissues themselves. *Henneguya pinnae* has been reported from *Ctenopoma kingsleyae* of West Africa. There are many other genera of Myxosporideans.

The Microsporidea contains a few genera, but only one important one, *Pleistophora* (also called *Plistophora*). There are a number of species of *Pleistophora* parasitizing freshwater and marine fishes. This genus is very close to *Ichthyosporidium*. *Pleistophora hyphessobryconis* parasitizes the tissues of many species of tetras and dwarf cichlids, and has little or no effective host specificity. As do other microsporideans, it causes cellular enlargement and cellular multiplication, as well as opacity of the tissues. The tissues eventually are killed. *Pleistophora* is the cause of neon tetra disease. The cysts are quite large, and best distinguished with the periodic acid/schiff staining technique (PA/S), a technique beyond the ability of aquarists.

Another Microsporidean, *Ichthyosporidium*, is also best diagnosed by this staining method. *Ichthyosporidium* has often been confused with the fungus, *Ichthyophonus*. This parasite probably occurs in more aquarium fishes than have been examined for it.

Last, *Glugea* is another Microsporidean that causes enlargement of the host cells before killing them.

In summary, it is hopeless for the aquarist to try to identify species of sporozoa. Properly prepared blood smears, or preserved whole fishes should be sent to an expert for identification. These are all tissue parasites, and treatments are not available. As stated in the Introduction, most species have been recorded from game fishes, because the study of such fishes is relevant to the interests of certain government agencies. Until a comprehensive program gets under way hopefully at the new National Aquarium and Fisheries Center in Washington, D.C., aquarists are advised to preserve fishes and record data. This will be the foundation of a future science of parasitic aquariology.

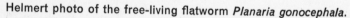

Helmert photo of the free-living flatworm *Planaria gonocephala*.

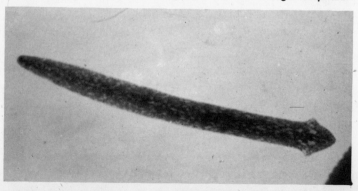

46

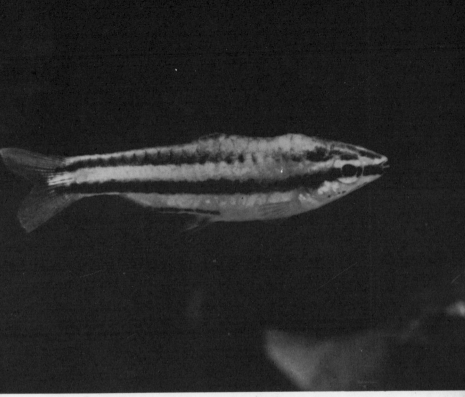

Zukal photo of *Nannostomus marginatus* with pleistophoriasis.

11. DIGENETIC FLUKES

Aquarists usually reserve the term *fluke* for certain flatworms found on the skin or gills of fishes. This usage is simplistic, and we must now begin our discussion by placing the term in broader perspective.

Phylum PLATYHELMINTHES = Flatworms
Class 1. TURBELLARIA   = Free-living planarians
Class 2. CESTOIDEA   = Tapeworms
Class 3. TREMATODA   = Flukes

And now we can subdivide the flukes into their taxonomic categories.

Subclass 1. ASPIDOGASTREA = Shield-worms
Subclass 2. DIGENEA   = Internal flukes
Subclass 3. MONOGENEA   = External flukes

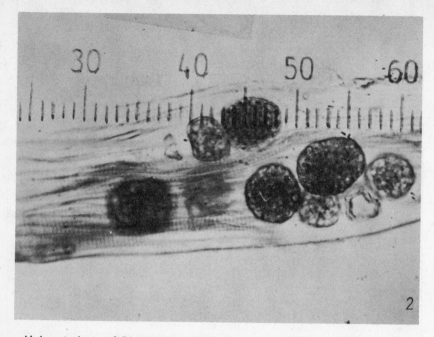

2

Helmert photo of *Pleistophora* within tissue of a fish; the numbers are microscope calibrations.

We are concerned with the *digenea*, or *digenetic trematodes*. I have called them internal flukes, because this is where they are most often found. What really distinguishes them from all other flukes, however, is their complex life cycle. This cycle is characterized by the phenomenon of *polyembryony with germinal lineage*. This term means that there is a multiplicity of twinning of the original fertilized egg (or *zygote*), but that this twinning occurs in delayed stages. Depending on the environment of the developing embryo, this embryo may become any of a number of things. All this will become clear as we go through a hypothetical life cycle.

The adult worm is a hermaphrodite (having both male and female reproductive systems) living in the intestine of the fish. There are others of its kind in the same location, and cross-fertilization is the rule. The eggs are fertilized, covered with a protective shell, and the shell is progressively hardened as it passes along the uterus toward the *uterine pore* to the outside of the worm. Now it is free in the intestine, is swept along with food and wastes and is evacuated with the wastes of the fish into the water. After a short time, the embryo within the egg is ready to hatch. A lid on the eggshell lifts open as the baby "worm" struggles to get out. The "worm" is free! This stage doesn't look like a worm at all, but like a little protozoan. It has a group of plates, each plate covered with *cilia,* enabling it to swim. The swimming larva is called a *miracidium.* If we look inside the miracidium we can see a number of simple structures, including some *penetration glands* and some little clusters of nuclei called *germ balls.* In the eggshell, what happened was that multiple twinning of the embryo took place. One of these embryos developed into our miracidium, and the rest were retained in the form of germ balls. These will be used later.

The swimming miracidium seeks out a proper species of snail, probably by smell. Finding one, it bores into the soft snail flesh, shedding its ciliated plates in the process, and elongating and enlarging within the snail, as it absorbs nourishment from the snail juices. The larva is now called a *sporocyst.* Some of the germ balls now begin to develop into another kind of larva. This next kind is characterized by a definite (although small) intestine, and

Cercariae of a *Dicrocoelium* genus of trematode, with long tails adequately fitting them for swimming. Knaack photo.

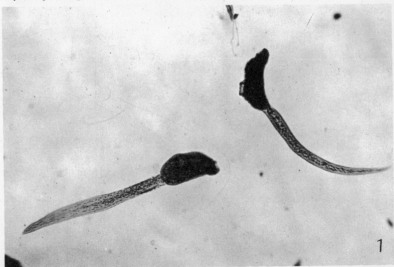

is termed the *redia* larva. The redia also has germ balls in it. There are many of these rediae produced by a single sporocyst, and they generally occur elsewhere in the snail. In fact, we assume that the rediae migrate to the snail's digestive gland, and begin chewing it up for nourishment. Finally, the germ balls in the rediae begin to form into other larvae. These other larvae have long tails, and work their way out of the redial parent, and out of the snail. These tailed larvae are called *cercariae*.

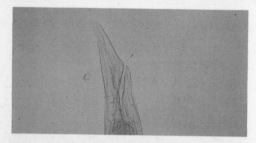

Tail end and anus of nematode from an *Epiplatys* from Togo; (below) its head end. Goldstein photos.

Tail end of a male nematode showing copulatory spicules. Goldstein photo.

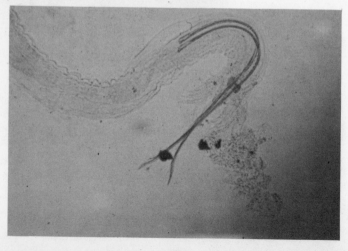

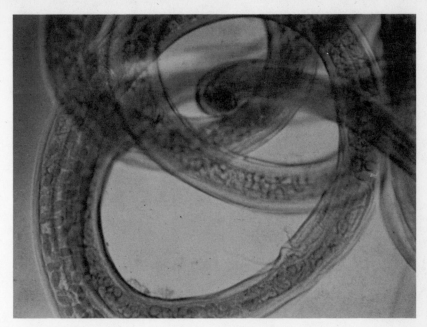

An egg-filled female nematode dissected from an elephantnose; (below) the nematode coiled up and encysted in this *Hyphessobrycon* was found to be longer than its host when removed and straightened out. Goldstein photos.

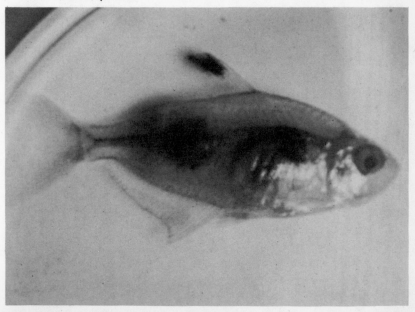

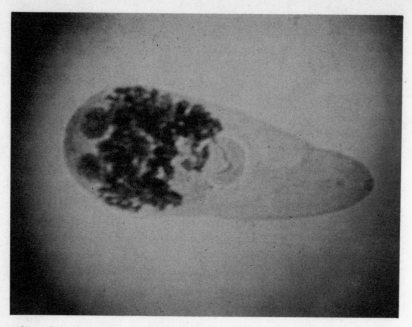

An adult digenetic trematode; noticeable is a sucker at the narrow (mouth) end, another in the center, the two testes at the bottom, and a mass of yolk-forming material in the lower half. Goldstein photo.

The cercaria swims out into the open, and may hang from the surface of the water or may immediately seek out a place to encyst. Let's assume it encysts in a small fish. Once encysted, it is called a *metacercaria*. Yellow grub and black spot are examples of metacercariae.

The small fish may have numerous cysts. Eventually it is eaten by a large fish, and the metacercariae break out of the cyst, migrate to the preferred area of the intestine, and mature, mate, and lay eggs. Thus, the cycle is completed.

There are many variations on this theme, mostly in terms of the final host and in the life cycle larval stages. But there are some principles too. First, the final host is a higher animal (fish, amphibian, reptile, bird, or mammal). Starting with a single miracidium from a single egg, we end up with many (often hundreds) of cercariae. Snails are almost always the first intermediate host. Altogether there may be three, four, or five hosts; but never less than two. Three is usual.

It is now clear why wild snails should never be kept in an aquarium with fishes. There is always the chance that they are infected and shedding cercariae. If you think that your wild snails are attractive, then you should set them up in jars with lettuce, let them breed, and use their offspring in your aquaria. The offspring will be "clean."

Adult flukes may exist in any part of the body of the host, depending on the species. There are digenea that infect the intestine, the stomach, eye, swim bladder, gall bladder, urinary system, heart, blood vessels, lymphatic system, or almost anywhere else. Metacercariae may encyst in the skin, muscles, mesenteries, or peritoneum. There are even some that preferentially encyst in the heart muscle. And there are some that don't encyst, but wander through the tissues (*mesocercariae*). Or, this stage may be bypassed, the cercaria penetrating the final host and developing directly to an adult worm. The variations are astronomical.

Diagnosis of adult worms is usually not possible and treatment for adult worms is not warranted. Metacercariae are often visible as yellow lumps or blackish spots just under the skin of the fish.

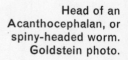
Head of an Acanthocephalan, or spiny-headed worm. Goldstein photo.

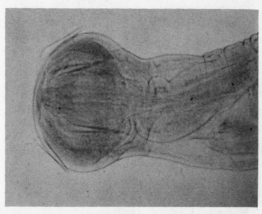

There are no drugs, but the metacercariae may be plucked out with a sterilized (flame, alcohol) needle. After picking them out, the wound should be swabbed with mercurochrome and the fish isolated until the wound heals. Unless the cysts are adjacent to the eye, or there are very many of them, it is advisable to leave them alone. These cysts will not multiply, and they do not grow very large. As such, the danger of damage is greater from the operation than from the disease. You may want to pick out one or two larger ones just for fun, and observe the living worms with your microscope or magnifying glass. In most cases, however, it is best to leave well enough alone. Understanding the disease will take away the fear of it.

12. DIGENETIC TREMATODES IN FISHES OF AQUARIUM INTEREST*

Parasite	Host	Site
Bucephalus barina	*Scatophagus argus*	intestine
Autorchis lintoni	*Astyanax fasciatus*	intestine
Heterorchis crumenifer	*Protopterus oethiopicus*	intestine
Emoleptalea synodontidos	*Synodontis notatus*	intestine
Callodistomum diaphanum	*Polypterus bichir*	gall bladder
Cholepotes ovofarctus	*Synodontis* sp.	gall bladder
Prosthenhystera obesa	*Leporinus, Xiphostoma*	gall bladder
Opisthorchis pedicellatus	*Mystus seenghala*	gall bladder
O. piscola	*Gymnarchus niloticus*	gall bladder
Phyllodistomum linguale	*G. niloticus*	urinary bladder
P. singhiai	*Mastacembelus armatus*	urinary bladder
P. spatulaeforme	*Malapterurus electricus*	urinary bladder
Gorgotrema barbius	*Barbus sarana*	urinary organ
Megacoelium plecostomi	*Hypostomus plecostomus*	stomach
Allocreadium chuscoi	*Aequidens pulcher*	intestine
A. wallini	*Crenicichla gaeyi*	intestine
A. singhi	*Barbus tor*	intestine
A. dollfusi	*Barbus tor*	intestine
A. hirnahi	*Barbus tor*	intestine
A. nakundi	*Barbus sarana*	intestine
A. sp.	*Mastacembelus* sp.	intestine
Procaudotestis uruguaensis	*Loricaria vetula*	stomach
Crepidostomum platense	*Pimelodus clarias*	intestine
Crassicutis cichlasomae	*Cichlasoma mayorum*	stomach
Eocreadium intermedium	*Plecostomus commersoni*	stomach
Creptotrema creptotrema	*Leporinus* sp.	intestine
Orientocreadium batrachoides	*Clarias batrachus*	intestine
O. barabankiae	*C. batrachus*	intestine
O. clariae	*C. batrachus*	intestine
O. mahendrai	*C. batrachus*	intestine

* This table and those to follow serve principally to emphasize the diversity of species in each group. Data for identification of species is beyond the scope of this book and in general would be of no practical value to the hobbyist.

O. vermai	C. batrachus, Mystus vittatus	intestine
O. hyderabadi	Ophiocephalus punctatus	intestine
O. philippai	O. punctatus	intestine
O. umadias	Clarias magur	intestine
Trematobrien haplochromios	Haplochromis moffati	intestine
Masenia collata	Clarias batrachus	intestine
M. dayali	C. batrachus	intestine
M. vittatusia	Mystus vittatus	intestine
M. gomtia	M. vittatus	intestine
Parspina bagre	Pimelodella metae	intestine
Proneochasmus argentinensis	Pimelodus clarius	intestine
Brientrema malapteruri	Malapterurus electricus, Distichodus lusosso	intestine
Genarchopsis faruquis	Mastacembelus armatus	intestine
Helostomatis helostomatis	Helostoma temmincki	stomach
Kalitrema kalitrema	Plecostomus punctatus	intestine
Microrchis megacotyle	Mylossoma aureum	intestine
Podocotyle aphanii	Aphanius mento	intestine
Pseudocladorchis cylindricus	Mylossoma aureum	intestine
P. macrostomus	Colossoma bidens	intestine
Acanthostomum gymnarchi	Gymnarchus niloticus	intestine
Sanguinicola argentinensis	Prochilodus platensis	heart
S. chalmersi	Auchenoglanis occidentalis	blood
Plagioporus nemachili	Aphanius mento	intestine
P. biliaris	Haplochromis flavii, Tilapia zillii	gall bladder
P. sp.	Tilapia sp.	intestine
Plehniella dentata	Clarias lazera	intestine

METACERCARIAE (GRUBS) IN FISHES OF AQUARIUM INTEREST

Euclinostomum vanderkuypi	Anabas testudineus	muscles
Neochasmus sp.	Aphanius mento	muscles
Euclinostomum heterostomum	Clarias sp.	throughout
Haplorchis sp.	Haplochromis flavii	skin, muscles
Transversotrema patialense	Macropodus cupanus	skin
Clonorchis sinensis	Tilapia spp.	muscles
Ascocotyle leighi	Cyprinodon variegatus	heart
A. angrense	Fundulus, Cyprinodon, Poecilia latipinna	blood vessels of gills
A. chandleri	C. variegatus, P. latipinna	blood sinuses of liver
A. tenuicollis	Gambusia affinis	heart
Tetracotyle-type Neascus	Epiplatys bitaeniatus	muscles, skin
Clinostomum-type	Aphyosemion lujae	muscle
Stictodora sclerogonocotyla	Tilapia galilaea	muscles

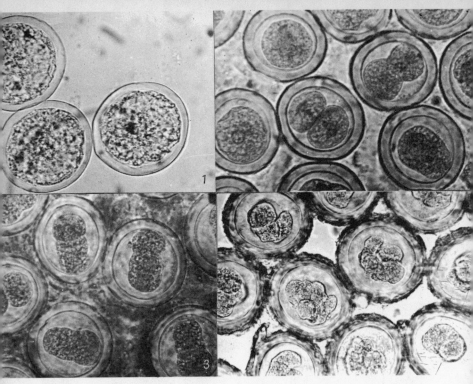

Helmert photos of nematode eggs: 1. unfertilized, 2. during first cellular division after fertilization, 3. cell division progressed, 4. after several cell divisions.

13. MONOGENETIC FLUKES

The MONOGENEA are a subclass of the Class TREMATODA of the Phylum PLATYHELMINTHES. Although parasitologists refer to all of the trematodes as *flukes*, aquarists have generally restricted the term to the monogenea.

Monogenea are primarily parasites of the skin and gills of all kinds of fishes. There are monogenea that occur in some strange places as well, e.g., the bladders of turtles and amphibians, and even the eye of the hippopotamus. All the monogenea of aquarium interest, of course, occur in the normal places, except for *Enterogyrus cichlidarum*, which lives, uniquely, in the intestine of fishes.

Monogenea are often rather small, requiring a magnifying glass for observation. They are hermaphrodites, and almost all genera are egg-layers. [*Gyrodactylus* is a live-bearer of sorts, but the nature of its reproductive system is still a mystery.] The head end may have lobes, and there may be a couple of pairs of eyes. The rear end serves for attachment, is generally enlarged, either elongated or flanged, and may have suckers, hooks, anchors, clamps, or a combination.

In nature, these animals show some degree of host-specificity, and there may be many species of one genus on a single species of host. This specificity is rather loose, however, and in the aquarium one may rapidly have an epidemic of flukes.

The life cycle is direct, requiring no intermediate hosts. Thus, the direct cycle combined with loose specificity makes epidemics not only possible, but rather frequent. Unfortunately, infection with a large number of flukes will cause the fish considerable irritation. This can be of the gills or the skin (according to the species of fluke), and there can be itching, scratching and bleeding. Fluke infections can be fatal.

A simple remedy for flukes is the use of formalin. Two drops per gallon generally will clear up the infection, but you may prefer to use up to four drops per gallon; this can be done gradually, always watching the fishes for signs of formalin-induced irritation. Flukes are extremely sensitive to this drug.

Several protozoan infections of the skin will cause the same symptoms. They are also susceptible to the drug, and so the aquarist can treat the tank on the basis of symptoms, rather than on carrying the diagnosis all the way to the finding of the pathogenic organism.

14. MONOGENEA FROM FISHES OF AQUARIUM INTEREST

Parasite	Host	Locality
Gyrodactylus cyprinodontii	*Epiplatys fasciatus*	Ghana
G. bullatarudis	*Poecilia reticulata*	Aquarium
G. cichlidarum	*Tilapia* spp., *Hemichromis fasciatus*, *H. bimaculatus*	Ghana
G. cytophagusi	*Aplocheilichthys gambianus*	Ghana
Metagyrodactylus indicus	*Argulus* sp. *on Ophiocephalus marulius*	West Bengal
Macrogyrodactylus polypteri	*Polypterus senegalis*	Gambia
M. clarii	*Clarias* spp.	Africa
M. congolensis	*Clarias* spp.	Africa

Dactylogyrus calbasi	*Labeo calbasi*	India
D. afrobarbae	*Barbus* spp.	Ghana
D. cauverii	*B. dubius*	India
D. chagunionis	*B. chagunio*	India
D. gussevi	*B. stigma*	India
D. kontii	*Labeo kontius*	India
D. longicirrus	*Barbus ticto, B. stigma*	India
D. moorthyi	*B. ticto, B. puckelli*	India
D. orientalis	*B. stigma*	India
D. puntii	*B. lateristriga*	Java
D. seenghali	*Mystus seenghala*	India
D. tripathi	*Barbus ticto, B. stigma*	India
Neodactylogyrus calbasi	*Labeo calbasu*	India
N. indicus	*Barbus stigma*	India
N. spinicirrus	*B. altianalis*	Uganda
Bifurcohaptor indicus	*Mystus vittatus*	India
Cichlidogyrus arthraçanthus	*Tilapia zillii*	Israel
C. tiberianus	*T. zillii*	Israel
C. bychowskii	*Hemichromis bimaculatus,*	
	H. fasciatus	Ghana
C. cirratus	*Tilapia galilaea*	Israel
C. tilapiae	*T. busumama, T. nilotica,*	
	T. galilaea	Israel
C. dionchus	*T. galilaea, Hemichromis*	
	fasciatus	Ghana
C. longicirrus	*H. fasciatus*	Ghana
Daitreosoma parvum	*Ambassis miops*	Guadalcanal
Heteroncocleidus bushkieli	*Macropodus opercularis*	Aquarium
Palombitrema heteroancistrium	*Astyanax fasciatus*	Costa Rica
Afrogyrodactylus characinis	*Micralestes* sp.	Ghana
Diplozoon barbi	*Barbus tetrazona,*	
	B. semifasciolatus	Aquarium
D. ghanense	*Alestes macrolepidotus*	Ghana
D. tetragonopterini	*Ctenobrycon spilurus,*	
	Gymnocorymbus ternetzi	Aquarium
Ancyrocephalus synodontii	*Synodontis victoriae*	Uganda
A. salinus	*Aphanius dispar*	Israel
Schilbetrema quadricornis	*Schilbe mystus*	Uganda
S. acornis	*S. mystus*	Uganda
Characidotrema elongata	*Alestes nurse*	Uganda
Quadriacanthus clariadis	*Clarias mossambica*	Uganda
Jainus jainus	*Chalceus macrolepidotus*	Brazil
J. robustus	*Creatochanes affinis*	Brazil
Unilatus brittani	*Plecostomus* sp.	Brazil
Urocleidoides carapus	*Gymnotus carapo*	Brazil
U. gymnotus	*G. carapo*	Brazil

U. microstomus	Hemigrammus microstomus	Brazil
U. stictus	Hyphessobrycon stictus	Brazil
U. virescens	Eigenmannia virescens	Brazil
Anacanthorus anacanthorus	Serrasalmus nattereri	Aquarium
A. brazilensis	S. nattereri	Aquarium
A. neotropicalis	S. nattereri	Aquarium
Cleidodiscus chavarriai	Rhamdia rogersi	Costa Rica
C. travassosi	R. rogersi	Costa Rica
C. amazonensis	Serrasalmus nattereri	Aquarium
C. piranhus	S. nattereri	Aquarium
C. serrasalmus	S. nattereri	Aquarium
C. costaricensis	Astyanax fasciatus	Costa Rica
C. strombicirrus	A. fasciatus	Costa Rica
C. microcirrus	Hemiodus semitaeniatus	Amazon
Gussevia spiralocirra	Pterophyllum scalare	Aquarium
G. minuta	Poecilia reticulata	Aquarium
Urocleidus orthus	Serrasalmus nattereri	Aquarium
U. crescentis	S. nattereri	Aquarium
U. cavanaughi	Aequidens maroni	Guyana
U. aequidens	A. maroni	Guyana
Diaccessorius anoculus	Plecostomus bolivianus	Bolivia
Monocleithrum lavergneae	Hemiodus semitaeniatus	Amazon
Enterogyrus cichlidarum	Tilapia zillii, T. nilotica	Israel
Onchobdella voltensis	Hemichromis fasciatus	Ghana
O. aframae	H. fasciatus	Ghana
O. spiricirra	H. bimaculatus	Ghana
O. pterygialis	H. bimaculatus	Ghana
O. krachii	Pelmatochromis guentheri	Ghana

Knaack photo of *Diplozoon*, a monogenetic fluke parasitic on gills, but rare in aquarium fishes.

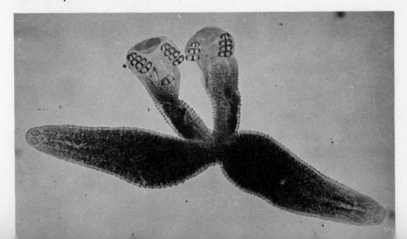

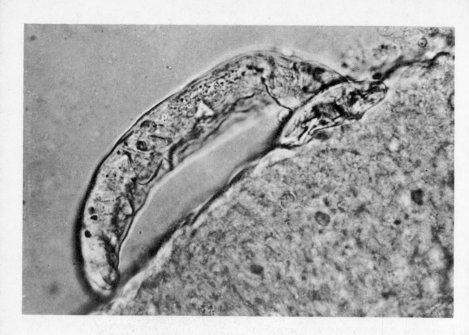

Dactylogyrus species gill flukes. Schubert photos.

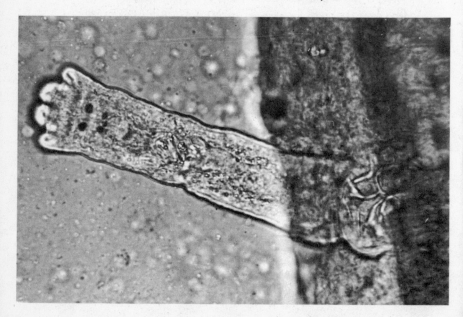

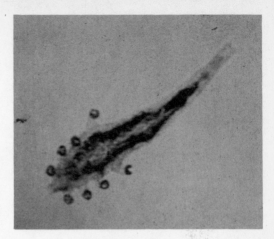

Monogenetic trematode, showing clamps at the ends of its divided attachment organ; Goldstein photo.

Saprolegnia or *Achyla* (fungi) growing on angelfish eggs; inset shows growth on a single egg; the large spheres are bubbles and the small ones spores. Photos: Zukal and (inset) by Emmens.

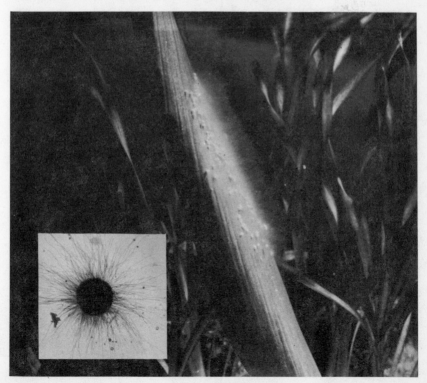

15. TAPEWORMS

Tapeworms are of practically no importance among aquarium fishes. As such, we will dispense with them rather quickly. Occasionally the marine aquarist who keeps small elasmobranch fishes (little sharks or rays) may notice small white, sometimes mobile, worm-like bits on the bottom of the aquarium, usually a millimeter or a little larger in size. These are the shed segments of marine tapeworms, and their appearance in the aquarium is not unusual. Neither should they be of any concern to the marine aquarist, as these tapeworms do no harm.

Tapeworms are classified as follows:

Phylum   PLATYHELMINTHES
Class   CESTOIDEA
Subclass EUCESTODA

Adult worms mostly:

Orders:		
PROTEOCEPHALA	In fishes, amphibians, reptiles.
TETRAPHYLLIDEA	In elasmobranch fishes.
LECANICEPHALA	In elasmobranch fishes.
TRYPANORHYNCHA	In elasmobranch fishes.
CYCLOPHYLLIDEA	In birds and mammals.
PSEUDOPHYLLIDEA	In fishes (sometimes mammals).
CARYOPHYLLIDEA	In fishes and tubificids.
SPATHEBOTHRIDEA	In (often primitive) fishes.
APORIDEA	In birds.
NIPPOTAENIIDEA	In fishes.
DISCULICEPITIDEA	In elasmobranch fishes.

Several of these orders are quite small, containing few species. The orders from elasmobranchs are essentially irrelevant to aquarists, and a few photographs of their attachment (or front) ends will suffice to illustrate their typical form. Only the Proteocephalans, Pseudophyllideans, and Caryophyllideans are of interest to aquarists.

Tapeworms vary from almost microscopic to many feet in length. Probably most of them fall between a quarter inch and four inches in total length. The front or attachment end is called the *scolex*. It may be of varying shapes and sizes, with suckers, hooks, tentacles, thorns, pads, or none of these. It may have outgrowths (*bothridia*) or depression-like grooves (*bothria*). Immediately behind the scolex is the growing region, where segments (divisions in the body) and *proglottids* (sets of genital organs) are formed. Usually, each segment contains one proglottid. As new segments are added, the older ones are pushed toward the rear, all the while growing and maturing, and eventually deteriorating. The business of a segment's proglottid is to produce fertilized eggs. In many tapeworms these eggs are shed as they are produced, while in others the eggs are retained in continually enlarging uterine organs. In either case, the oldest segments are eventually shed from the worm.

The adult (sexually active) tapeworm lives in the intestine of its host. Thus, as eggs or segments are shed, they are pushed down the intestinal canal and eventually evacuated with the host's solid wastes.

The life cycles of relatively few kinds of tapeworms are known. In general, however, it is thought that the eggs hatch in water to release a ciliated larva looking much like a protozoan. This little larva is eaten by a small crustacean, such as *Cyclops* or *Daphnia*, and develops in the crustacean's hemocoel (or blood sinus or blood cavity). The crustacean is next eaten by a small fish, and the larva develops a stage further in the fish's muscles, peritoneum, or mesenteries. The small fish is next eaten by the original type of fish, and the larva now matures in the intestine, grows, and begins to produce eggs. The host in which sexual activity occurs is the *definitive host*; all other hosts are called *intermediate hosts*. The cycle just outlined may be abbreviated, extended, or totally different, depending on the type of tapeworm. But this was a good, *average* cycle of a fish tapeworm.

Tapeworms really do no harm except in unusual cases. The adult worm is content to wander about its selected area of intestine, mating with other tapeworms or with itself, and feeding by means of microscopic brush-like projections from its body surface. It has been occupying a parasitic habit for so many eons, that there is no trace of a digestive system. Instead, it lets the host carry on most of the digestion and competes with the host for the broken-down molecules. A healthy host can support many small or one large (according to species) tapeworm(s). A starving host will expel its tapeworms. Larval tapeworms in small fishes, however, may do some damage by their shear numbers and the amount of nutrient they require. They cannot be expelled, as they are

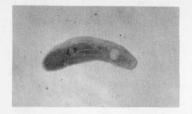

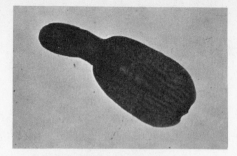

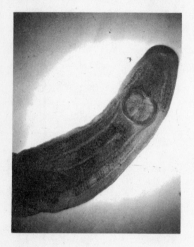

The broad front end of the metacercaria above makes it a diplostomulum type of larva; (left) two magnifications of a yellow grub-type metacercaria, and (below) section through a mass of metacercariae, each cyst containing a single parasite; triangular canal is intestine. Goldstein photos.

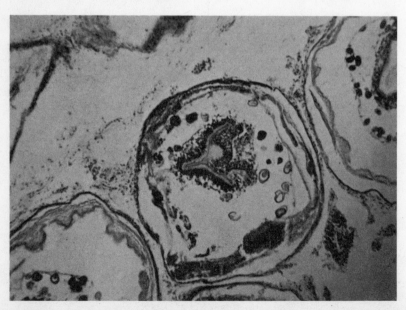

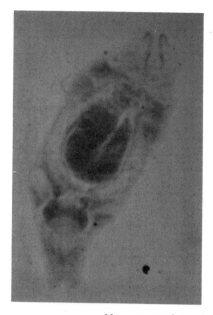
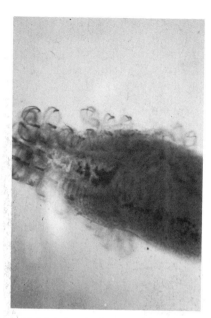

Monogenea from fishes. Goldstein photos.

usually encapsulated, and even if they aren't, their location eliminates any chance of escape from the host. In general, their presence cannot be determined except at autopsy. In any case, they are unusual in aquarium fishes, and the damage to fishes in general from larval tapeworms in general is too insignificant for the aquarist to worry about.

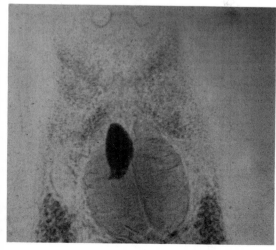

Head of monogenetic trematode. Goldstein photo.

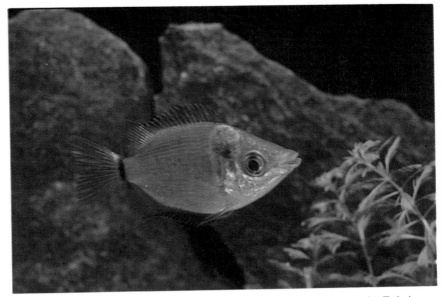

Bacterial skin infection following a wound, *Helostoma temmincki*. Zukal photo.

Imported fishes undergo considerable stress from capture and storage and crowding, are usually underfed if fed at all, and may be expected to have expelled any tapeworms they once may have had in their intestines. Thus, considering the life cycles, the rarity of infection, the difficulty of diagnosis, the lack of damage, etc., the aquarist can safely forget about treating tapeworms. Even when they occur, they are very good parasites, doing practically no damage to their hosts.

Elasmobranch fishes are almost 100% infected with Tetraphyllideans and Trypanorhynchs. Teleosts are rarely infected, and then most often with Pseudophyllideans, less often with Proteocephalans. The Holostean fish *Amia calva* is infected with a very rare type of primitive Pseudophyllidean, as well as with other things. Other Holostean fishes (gars) are also of considerable interest. Chondrostean fishes (sturgeons, paddle fishes) are not usually kept in aquaria. In short, each evolutionary line of fishes may be host to an evolutionary line of tapeworms, and the parasites seem to have evolved along with their hosts.

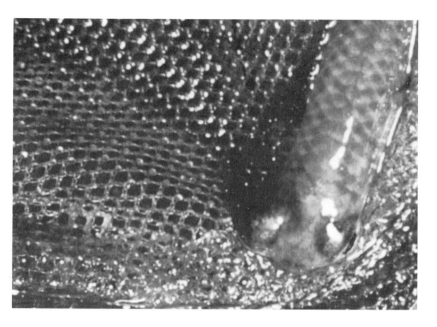

Austrofundulus dolichopterus with exophthalmia (pop-eye). Goldstein photo.

Zukal photo of *Nematocentrus macculochi* with bacterial skin infection following a wound.

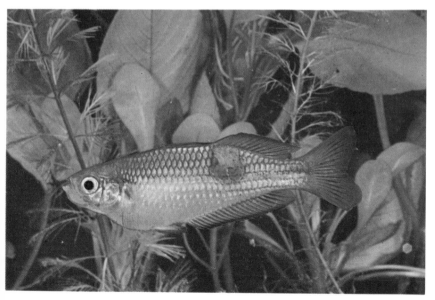

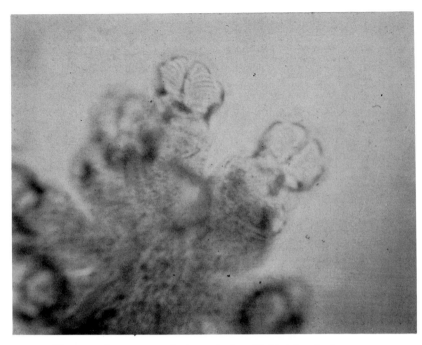

Clamps of monogenetic trematodes. Goldstein photos.

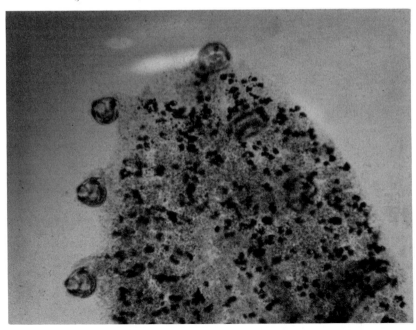

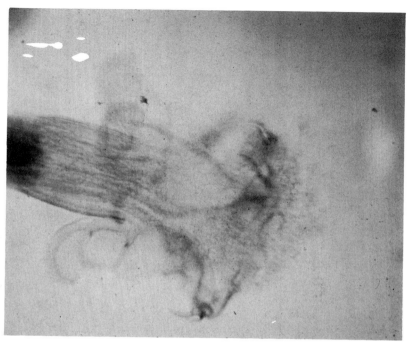

Scolices (heads) of marine tapeworms from rays. Goldstein photos.

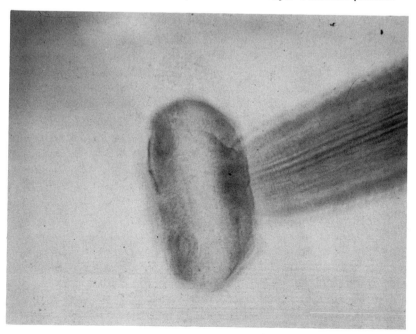

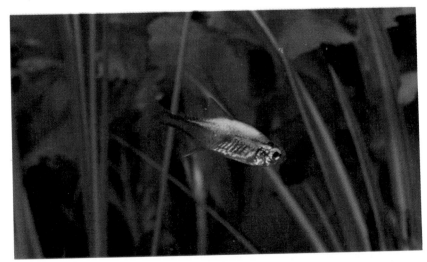

Protozoan infection, probably pleistophoriasis, in muscle tissue of a neon tetra.

Pelvicachromis species with congenital absence of tail. Zukal photo.

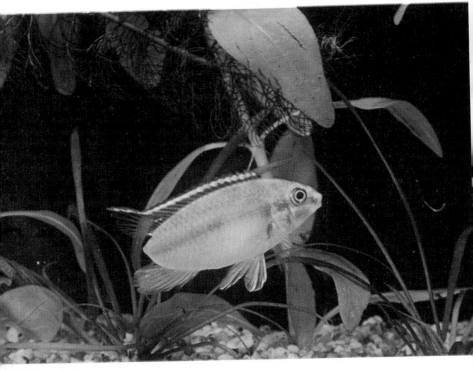

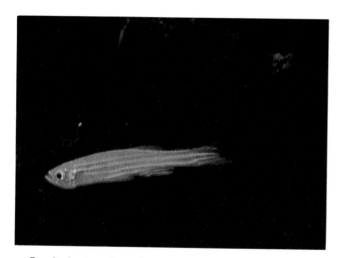

Brachydanio rerio suffering from old age and loss of appetite. Zukal photo.

Hemigrammus gracilis with *Saprolegnia* invasion of a head wound. Zukal photo.

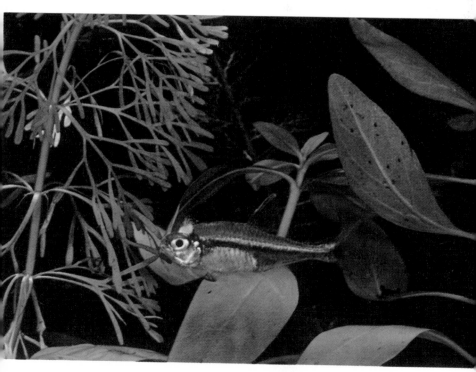

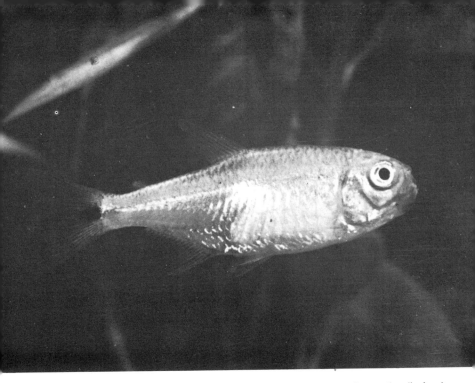

Hyphessobrycon scholzei with bacterial destruction of mouth; (below) *Puntius (Barbus) stoliczkanus* with hollow bellies, possibly indicating tuberculosis. Zukal photos.

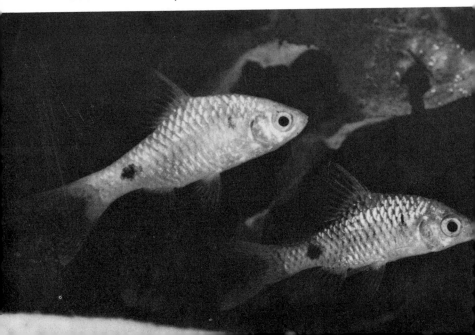

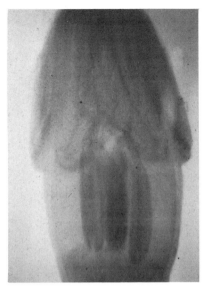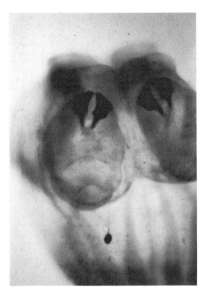

Scolices (heads) of marine tapeworms from sharks. Goldstein photos.

Aquarists in any part of the United States can have an excellent local society program on diseases, especially if tapeworms are used as a living demonstration. Because Proteocephalans are the most constant in form, are simple, large, and easily found in large salamanders, frogs, reptiles, and some fishes, they are ideal animals for a program. There is no comparison between seeing living and preserved (or just photographed) material.

No attempt should be made to purge aquarium fishes of tapeworms. And no attempt should be made to kill larval tapeworms in their tissues.

An exceptional form is *Ligula intestinalis*, a member of the order Pseudophyllidea. As an adult, it may be found in diving and wading birds in Europe, and in mergansers in the United States. It lives only briefly in birds, attaining almost complete size and development in the prior intermediate host. This intermediate host may be any of a number of freshwater fishes, including catfish, minnows, bass, salmon, perch, and sticklebacks. The last larval stage lives and grows in the body cavity (not the gut!) of the fish, in which it may grow so large as to cause great swelling of the fish. When the bird eats the fish, the worm quickly segments, matures, fills with eggs, and is expelled.

Similar to *Ligula* is the Pseudophyllidean, *Schistocephalus solidus*. Again, the larvae may be found in sticklebacks, sculpins or trout. In the stickleback, of course, it may cause great enlargement of the body cavity. Adults are in fish-eating birds.

Because of the dependence on birds and crustaceans for the completion of the life cycle, these worms can cause no epidemics in aquaria. Any aquarist finding either of these infections in native fish aquaria should preserve the fish after slitting its belly with a razor blade. If the enlarged abdomen was due to tapeworm infestation, the worms will pop out.

Amia calva, the bowfin, dogfish or mudfish, is widely distributed throughout the United States, and its young stages are considered very desirable aquarium fishes by connoisseurs. Examination of the gut of larger specimens will yield *Proteocephalus ambloplitis* (which ordinarily is found in basses), a Proteocephalan worm. Occasional fish will also yield specimens of the ancient and primitive Pseudophyllidean, *Haplobothrium globuliforme*. The

Pelvicachromis pulcher with clinostomiasis (yellow grub) above the eye. Zukal photo.

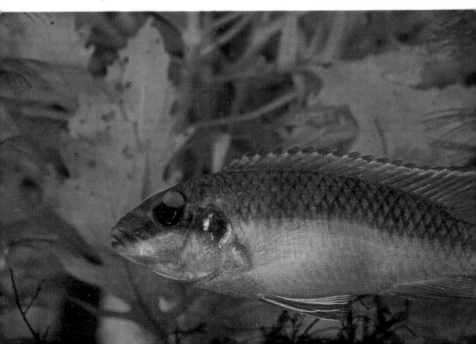

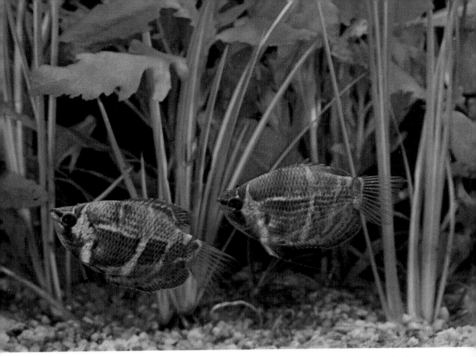

Sphaerichthys osphromenoides with bacterial skin infections. Zukal photo.

scolex of this worm resembles, superficially only, the scolex of a Trypanorhynch tapeworm, in that it has four tentacles. However, in Trypanorhynchs the tentacles are eversible and are armed with many rose thorn-shaped hooks. *Haplobothrium* also forms false scolex-like attachment organs, where the body of the tapeworm has broken.

Occasional specimens of *Tubifex* and *Limnodrila* worms (and other related worms, all called "tubifex" by aquarists), may be infected with unusual tapeworms of the Order Caryophyllidea. These tapeworms occur as adults in the gut of suckers (*Catastomus*) and minnows, as well as in tubificid worms. Apparently the finding of specialized tapeworms in annelid worms is an adaptation wherein the larval stage of the tapeworm has achieved success by maturing precociously. Not only are the Caryophyllideans unusual in their hosts; they are also unusual in their form. They are not segmented and have only a single proglottid (set of reproductive organs).

They may also occur in some fishes of aquarium interest. Species of *Wenyonia* have been found in *Synodontis* and *Chrysichthys* in the Sudan and Sierra Leone. *Lytocestoides tanganyikae* occurs in *Alestes* sp. *Lytocestus* occurs in siluroid and mormyrid fishes. *Stocksia* is from *Clarias* in Sierra Leone, and *Djombangia* is reported from *Clarias* in Java.

Below and opposite page: Zukal photos of *Macropodus opercularis* with exophthalmia (pop-eye).

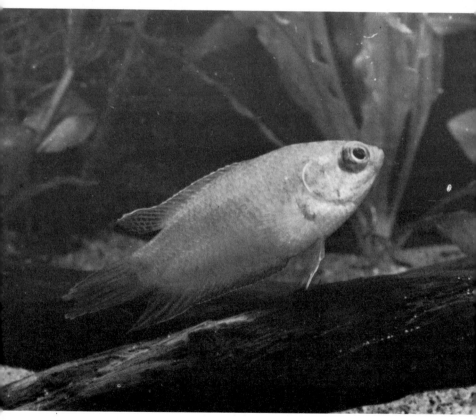

Among the Proteocephala, *Marsypocephalus* was reported from siluroids in the Nile and from *Clarias* in Lake Tanganyika. *Monticellia* occurs in some siluroids from the Amazon drainage. *Peltidocotyle* was found in *Platystoma tigrinum* of the Amazon. *Ephedrocephalus* is from *Phractocephalus*, another Amazon fish. And there are many, many more.

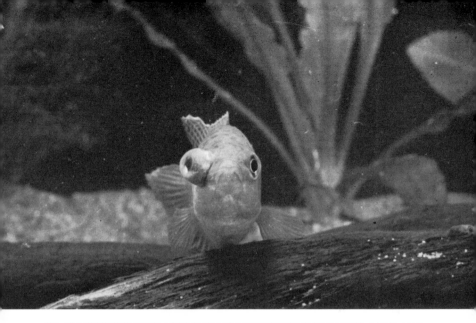

16. TAPEWORMS WHOSE DEFINITIVE HOSTS ARE OF AQUARIUM INTEREST
Order PROTEOCEPHALA

Parasite	Host	Locality
Marsypocephalus rectangularus	*Heterobranchus anguillaris*	Egypt (Nile)
M. davyi	*H. bidorsalis*	Sierra Leone
M. heterobranchus	*H. bidorsalis*	Nile
M. tanganyikae	*Clarias lazera*	Tanganyika
Monticellia lenha	*Platystomatichthys sturio*	Amazon
M. megacephala	*P. sturio*	Amazon
M. piracatinga	*Pimelodus pati*	Amazon
M. piramutab	*Brachyplatystoma vaillanti*	Amazon
M. rugosa	*Pseudoplatystoma fasciatus*	Amazon
M. spinulifera	*P. fasciatus*	Amazon
M. sorubim	*Sorubim lima* (?)	Amazon
Peltidocotyle rugosa	*Platystoma tigrinum*	Amazon
P. myzofera	*Platystomatichthys sturio*	Amazon
Rudolphiella lobosa	*Pimelodus pati*	Paraguay
Ephedrocephalus microcephalus	*Pharctocephalus hemiliopterus*	Amazon
Endorchis piraeeba	*Brachyplatystoma filamentosum*	Amazon
Electrotaenia malopteruri	*Malopterurus electricus*	Africa
Megathylacus jaudia	*Rhamdia* sp.	Brazil
Zygobothrium megacephalum	*Phractocephalus hemiliopterus, Pirara bicolor*	Amazon

Parasite	Host	Locality
Nomimoscolex piraeeba	*Brachyplatystoma filamentosum*	Amazon
N. kaparari	*Pseudoplatystoma tigrinum*	Amazon
N. sudobim	*P. fasciatum*	Amazon
N. lenha	*Platystomatichthys sturio*	Amazon
N. piracatinga	*Pimelodus pati*	Amazon
Corallobothrium solidum	*Malopterurus electricus*	Africa
Proteocephalus bivitellatus	*Tilapia* sp.	Sierra Leone
P. cunningtoni	*Dinopterus cunningtoni*	L. Tanganyika
P. dinotopteri	*Dinopterus cunningtoni*	L. Tanganyika
P. fossatus	*Pimelodus pati*	Paraguay
P. glanduliger	*Clarias anguillaris*	Egypt
P. kuyukuyu	*Pseudodoras niger*	Brazil
P. macrophallus	*Cichla monoculus*	Brazil
P. microscopius	*C. ocellaris*	Brazil
P. pentastoma	*Polypterus bichir*	Sudan
P. sulcatus	*P. endlichi*	Sudan
P. synodontis	*Synodontis schall*	Nile
P. beauchampi	*S. schall*	Sudan

Order CARYOPHYLLIDEA

Caryophyllaeus laticeps	*Barbus, Nemacheilus,* etc.	
C. acutus	*Clarias batrachus*	Java
C. javanicus	*C. batrachus*	Java
C. microcephalus	*C. batrachus*	Java
C. oxycephalus	*C. batrachus*	Java
C. tenuicollis	*C. batrachus*	Java
C. chalmersius	*C. anguillaris*	Nile
Wenyonia virilis	*Synodontis schall*	Nile
W. nilotica	*S. schall*	Nile
W. acuminata	*S. membranaceus*	Nile
W. longicauda	*S. gambiensis*	Sierra Leone
Lytocestus adhaerens	*Clarias fuscus*	Hong Kong
L. alestesi	*Alestes nurse*	Sudan
L. burmanicus	*Clarias batrachus*	Sudan
L. indicus	*C. batrachus*	Sudan
L. parvulus	*C. batrachus*	Sudan
L. filiformis	*Mormyrus caschive*	Sudan
Bovienia serialis	*Clarias batrachus*	Java
Djombangia penetrans	*C. batrachus*	Java
Lytocestoides tanganyikae	*Alestes* sp.	Tanganyika
Monobothrioides cunningtoni	*Auchenoglanis orientalis*	Tanganyika
M. woodlandi	*Clarias mellandi*	Zambia
Stocksia pujehuni	*Clarias lazera*	Sierra Leone

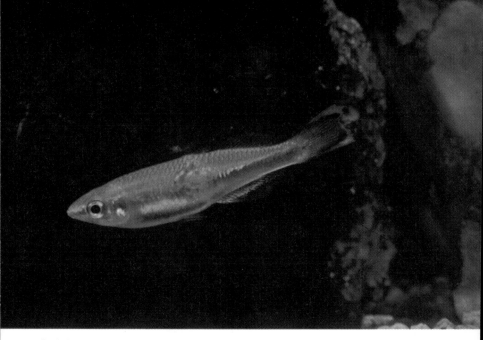

Bedotia geayi with bacterial invasion of a skin wound. Photo by R. Zukal.

Order PSEUDOPHYLLIDEA

Marsupimetra hastata	*Polyodon spathula*	North America
M. confusa	*P. spathula*	North America
M. parva	*P. spathula*	North America
Bothriocephalus musculosus	*Aequidens portalegrensis*	Aquarium
Haplobothrium globuliforme	*Amia calva*	North America
H. bistrobilae	*Amia calva*	North America
Polyoncobothrium polypteri	*Polypterus bichir*	Egypt
P. ciliotheca	*Clarias anguillaris*	Egypt
P. clarias	*C. anguillaris*	Egypt, Sudan
P. cylindraceum	*C. anguillaris*	Egypt, Sudan
P. fulgidum	*C. anguillaris*	Egypt, Sudan
P. gordoni	*Heterobranchus bidorsalis*	Sierra Leone
Senga besnardi	*Betta splendens*	Thailand
S. lucknowensis	*Mastacembelus armatus*	India
S. ophiocephalina	*Ophiocephalus argus*	China
	O. striatus	India
S. pycnomera	*O. marulius*	India
S. malayana	*O. striata*	Malaya
S. filiformis	*O. micr̓opeltes*	Malaya
S. parva	*O. micropeltes*	Malaya
S. sp.	*Aplocheilus panchax* (encysted larva)	Malaya

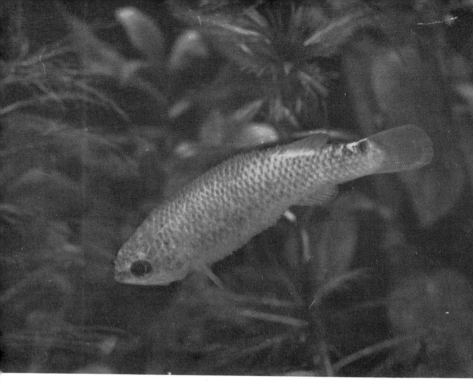

Above and below   Zukal photos of *Rivulus cylindraceus* suffering from dropsy; any of several Gram-negative bacteria may be responsible for the fluid-filled tissues causing the external appearance.

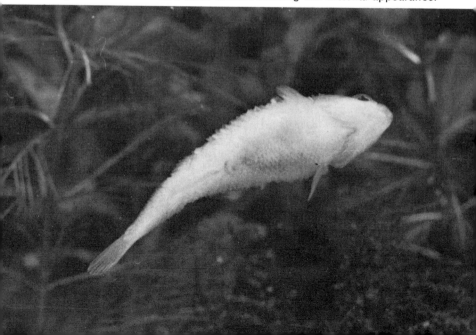

17. ROUNDWORMS

The Phylum ASCHELMINTHES contains a number of Classes, including the Class NEMATODA, the roundworms. There are about half a million species of nematodes, and they occupy all types of habitats, from soil to ocean depths to arctic ice. Most of them are free-living forms, and play an important role in the biology of soil and the health of plants. Parasitism has arisen many times in independent lines of nematodes. And so, there are no generalizations that can be made about parasitic nematodes. Rather, our generalizations apply to the Class itself.

Most nematodes are typically worm-shaped, but some are short and blunt, while others are very filamentous. The body wall contains a single layer of longitudinal muscle, and this means that nematodes can contract lengthwise, but not laterally. Their total length, therefore, cannot shrink; the worms can only coil, much like a watch spring. They range from microscopic to several feet in length. Some examples of roundworms you may have heard of are: microworms, vinegar eels, trichina worms (from eating uncooked pork), elephantiasis (a rare, late stage of human infection with any of several roundworms), dog heartworm and hookworms. There are many, many others.

As you might expect from their very numbers, roundworms may infect any part of the body. Many of them can exist in a variety of hosts and host-specificity is very low in the group as a whole. A single species of roundworm may not only exist in a variety of animals, but also in a variety of locations within any one of them.

Nematodes have a complete intestine. Food goes in one end and out the other. The mouth may be armed with cutting tools. The sexes are separate; males are generally smaller than females. The females may lay eggs (**oviparous**), or retain the eggs until hatching and thence release larvae (ovoviviparous). There are a series of molts required before the nematode is sexually mature. Some nematodes are parasites all during their lives, others only as adults, and still others only as larvae. They parasitize all classes of higher animals, all classes of invertebrates, and may be expected to be found anywhere. Aquarists are likely to encounter them in the body cavity or the intestine of fishes. Parasitic forms may

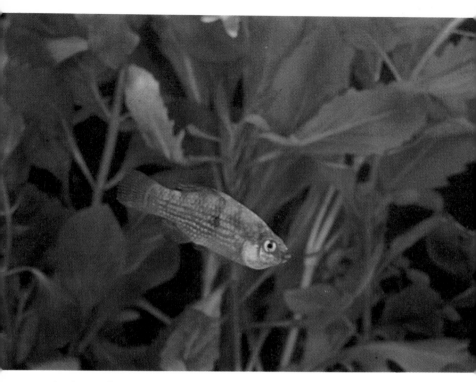

Jordanella floridae with hollow belly, the causes of which are many and varied. Zukal photo.

require many, one, or no intermediate hosts. The reproductive systems are unusual, though not complex. The sperm are amoeboid, lacking flagella.

Nematodes are difficult to identify, except by a specialist. Color, size, host, and general shape are not good criteria, because so few species have been identified with aquarium fishes, at least in the popular literature. If one finds them in a fish, they should be preserved in alcohol or formalin and mailed to a specialist for identification. The table of *nematodes from fishes of aquarium interest* is not complete, but only reflects a large part of what has been done so far. You will note that some genera of worms occur on different continents, while some are restricted to one continent.

But since I have omitted fish species (and localities) that are not of aquarium concern, some of these apparently one-continent genera are to be considered probably wider ranging.

Generally, mass infestations are of no concern to the aquarist, although they may occur in ponds. Various live foods may deliver potentially parasitic species to your fishes, but serious problems are rare. Even in situations where the aquarist has delivered many parasites to his fishes, the parasites seldom do much harm. Thus, treatment is not of concern to you.

Should you feel that treatment for roundworms is worth a try (perhaps you are losing some newly imported fishes for no apparent reason, or perhaps you found roundworms in one of the carcasses you examined), then use the following procedure. At your pet dealer's rack for dog and cat medicines, look for dog or cat food containing the drug *thiabendazole*. This is the newest and

Xiphophorus helleri near death; this condition is terminal to many diseases, poisonings, environmental factors, and dietary deficiencies. Zukal photo.

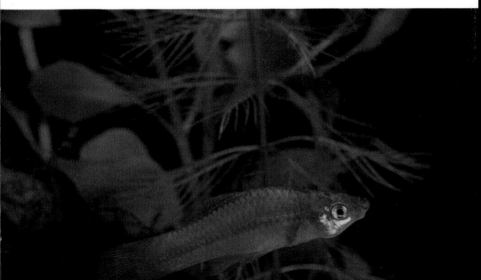

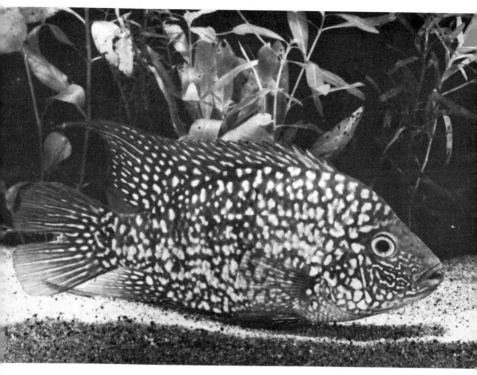

Early stage of tailrot in a generally healthy *Cichlasoma cyanoguttatum* that will probably recover spontaneously. Zukal photo.

mildest (as well as most effective) nematocide on the market. Just feed some of the drug-treated food to your suspected fish. If they have intestinal nematodes, the worms will probably be killed and expelled. The danger to such a drug is the ever-present danger of nematodes in a part of the body from which they cannot be expelled. In this case, the dead worms are more dangerous, locked in the host, than the live ones ever were. Thiabendazole is the only acceptable nematocide. The others are far more debilitating to the host, as many of them have arsenical or antimonial bases.

18. NEMATODES FROM FISHES OF AQUARIUM INTEREST

Parasite	Host	Locality
Capillaria fritschi	Malapterurus electricus	Egypt
C. minima	Leporinus sp.	Brazil
C. pterophylli	Pterophyllum scalare	South America
C. zederi	Hoplias malabaricus	Brazil
Rondonia rondoni	Pimelodus clarias,	
	Colossoma mitre	South America
Cosmoxynema vianai	Curimata gilberti	Brazil
Nematoxynema piscicola	Distichodus sp.	Cameroon
Travnema travnema	Curimata elegans	Brazil
Gendria tilapiae	Tilapia galilaea	Niger
Contracaecum collieri	Cyprinodon variegatus	Texas
Dujardinascaris cenotae	Rhamdia guatamalensis	Yucatan
D. malapteruri	Malapterurus electricus	Sudan
Hedrurus iheringi	Cynolebias bellottii	Argentina
H. orestiae	Orestias muelleri	L. Titicaca
Camallanus anabantis	Anabas testudineus,	
	Clarias batrachus,	
	Barbus filamentosus,	
	Ophiocephalus punctatus,	
	Rasbora daniconius	Asia
C. ophicephali	Ophiocephalus striatus	India, Thailand
C. trichogasterae	Trichogaster trichopterus	Thailand
C. unispiculus	Mastacembelus armatus	India
C. yehi	Ophiocephalus striatus	Singapore
C. longitridentatus	Clarias batrachus	Singapore
C. sp.	Aplocheilus panchax	India
Procamallanus laeviconchis	Synodontis schall	Egypt
P. amarali	Leporinus sp.	Brazil
P. cearensis	Astyanax bimaculatus	Brazil
P. fariasi	Leporinus sp.	Brazil
P. planoratus	Clarias batrachus,	
	Ophiocephalus spp.	Asia
P. wrighti	Astyanax sp.,	
	Hoplias malabaricus,	
	Leporinus sp.	Brazil
P. spiculogubernaculus	Clarias teysmanni	Ceylon
P. malaccensis	Ophiocephalus lucius	Asia
Cucullanus pinnai	Pimelodus clarias,	
	Pseudoplatystoma sp.	Brazil
Neocucullanus neocucullanus	Characidae	Brazil
Proleptus anabantis	Anabas testudineus	Thailand
Pseudoproleptus vestibulus	Mastacembelus armatus	India
Haplonema immutatum	Amia calva	Iowa

Rhabdochona sp.	*Clarias lazera*	Israel
R. acuminata	*Brycon* sp., *Barbus* spp.,	
	Pimelodella sp.	Brazil
R. kidderi	*Rhamdia guatamalensis*	Yucatan
Spinitectus asper	*Prochilodus scrofa*	Brazil
S. major	*Mastacembelus armatus*	India
S. mastacembeli	*M. armatus*	India
S. singhi	*M. armatus*	India
S. rudolphiheringi	*Pimelodella lateristriga*	Brazil
S. yorkei	*P. lateristriga*	Brazil
S. armatus	*Mystus tengara*	India
Philometra baylisi	*Pimelodus clarias*	Brazil
P. congolensis	*Clarias* sp.	Congo
P. senticosa	*Arapaima gigas*	Amazon

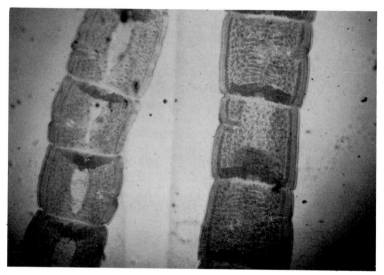

Segments of a *Proteocephalus* type of tapeworm from a freshwater fish. Goldstein photo.

Asymphylodora tincae	*Haplochromis flavii*	Israel
Paracamallanus cyathopharynx	*Clarias* sp.	North Africa
P. ophiocephali	*Ophiocephalus gachua*	India
Agamofilaria sp.	*Ophiocephalus striatus,*	
	Clarias batrachus	Thailand
Parastictodora sp.	*Aphanius mento* (larvae)	Israel
Zeylanema sp.	*Betta picta*	Asia
Z. kulasirii	*Anabas testudineus,*	
	Ophiocephalus	
	punctatus	Asia

86

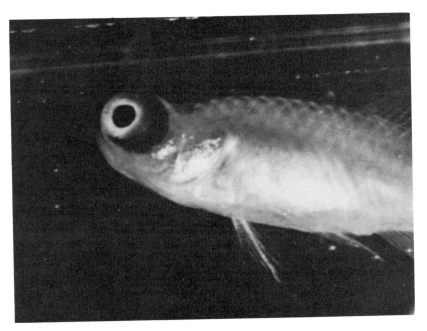

Pop-eye in *Austrofundulus dolichopterus*. Goldstein photo.

Infection of lateral line system of *Labeotropheus trewavasae*, probably caused by Gram-negative bacteria. Goldstein photo.

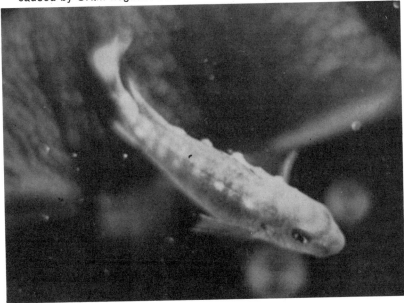

Z. sweeti	*Rasbora daniconius,* *Ophiocephalus* spp.	Asia
Z. anabantis	*Anabas testudineus,* *Rasbora daniconius,* *Ophiocephalus punctatus,* *Barbus filamentosus*	Asia
Z. pearsei	*Anabas testudineus,* *Rasbora daniconius*	Asia
*Gnathostoma spinigerum**	*Trichogaster microlepis,* *T. pectoralis, A. testudineus,* *C. batrachus*	Asia

19. THORNY-HEADED WORMS

The thorny-headed worms comprise their own phylum of animals. This means that we are unable to relate them to any other animals we know of. They are all parasites, undoubtedly of ancient origin. As with the tapeworms, the thorny-headed worms do not have a mouth or any trace of a digestive system. There is usually a two host life cycle, with the definitive host being a vertebrate animal, and the intermediate host being an arthropod. All classes of vertebrates are known to harbor these noxious parasites, but of course we are only concerned with the species that invade fishes.

The adult worm lives in the intestine of the fish. There are separate males and females. The reproductive system is unique and quite complex, involving an egg-sorting apparatus which determines the eggs to be retained and the eggs to be fertilized and shed. Although two hosts are usual, there are different stages within a single intermediate host. However, in some species of worms, three hosts may be normal to the life cycle.

The extraordinary apparatus which separates these worms from all other parasites is the single, protrusible, armed proboscis. This massive attachment organ is buried deep into the lining of the fish's gut and gut wall, and may cause considerable damage. Even in a light infection, one can feel the nodule of inflammatory tissue which forms about each of these invaded sites. One of the easiest ways to find thorny-headed worms without even slitting open the gut of the dead fish, is to pass the gut between your

* Ordinarily *G. spinigerum* is a parasite of fish-eating mammals. On occasion it infects man, and is discussed in every parasitology textbook.

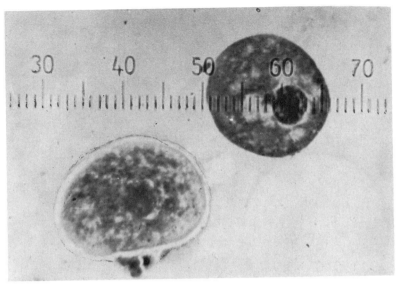

Chilodon(ella), perhaps *C. cyprini*; this protozoan parasite can cause skin discoloration, seen as light blotches. Helmert photo.

fingers for its whole length. You'll easily feel the bump of tissue where the proboscis of a worm is lodged, if the worm is any size at all worth considering. Sometimes, the proboscis of the worm breaks through the gut, and causes death in the same way a person can be killed by a bleeding ulcer or a ruptured appendix. Bacteria are normal to the gut contents, but as a result of a perforation in the gut, they get out into the tissues of the host and cause a general infection or *bacteremia*, as the blood carries them through the body.

The thorny-headed worms make up the Phylum Acanthocephala, which literally means "hooked heads." The shape of the proboscis, the shape and distribution of its hooks or spines, and internal considerations are all used in classification. It is a small phylum, archaic, and of considerable interest to biologists, who haven't the faintest idea of from what it could have originated.

There are several species in North American game and trash fishes, and it would be no trouble to find some specimens for a club program on diseases. Sunfish, basses, perch, and *Amia calva* are all infected. Sometimes one finds a thorny-headed worm that is a bright yellow or orange color, whereas most parasites are generally white. This coloration is due to ingested (actually absorbed, since they have no gut) fatty material from the host's gut. Thorny-headed worms may appear flat and segmented and thus be confused with tapeworms. This will quickly pass as the worms take up fluid and fatten so that they resemble roundworms more than anything else. They have no segments; some may have markings that resemble segments. In general, they are banana-shaped and tightly bound to the host's gut. They usually have to be cut out.

Infestation with thorny-headed worms is not a major problem in aquaria. You'd never know it if your fishes had a few worms in them. They are more a problem to hatcheries. Thus, there is no need to be concerned with treatment.

Acanthocephala are not especially host-specific as a group. Apparently the food habits of the fish are more important than its evolutionary pedigree.

Zukal photo of *Macropodus opercularis* with superficial and systemic bacteremia; the fish is beyond help and should be destroyed.

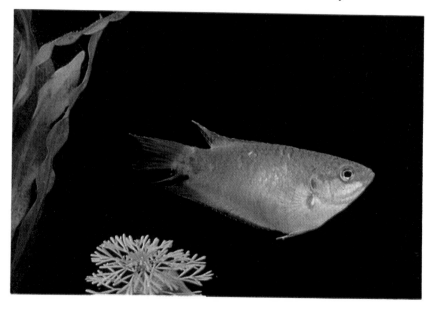

20. THORNY-HEADED WORMS FROM FISHES OF AQUARIUM INTEREST

Parasite	Host	Locality
Neoechinorhynchus australe	*Prochilodus platensis*	Uruguay
N. cylindratum	*Amia calva* and other fishes	North America
N. doryphorum	*Jordanella floridae,* *Fundulus majalis* (larvae), *F. parva* (larvae)	Florida
N. octonucleatum	*Therapon argenteus*	Philippines
N. spectabilis	*Curimata elegans*	Brazil
Hexaspiron nigericum	*Synodontis membranaceus*	Nigeria
Gracilisentis variabilis	*Hypostomus plecostomus,* *H. literatus,* *H. aureoguttatus,* *H. melanopterus*	Brazil
Pandosentis iracundus	*Aequidens pulcher,* *Crenicichla gaeyi*	Venezuela
Acanthogyrus acanthogyrus	*Labeo rohita*	India
Acanthodelta scorzai	Pimelodid catfish	Venezuela
Quadrigyrus torquatus	*Hoplias malabaricus,* *Crenicichla geayi,* *Astyanax bimaculatus,* *Gephyrocharax valenciae,* *Synbrachus marmoratus*	South America

Goldstein photo of *Aphyoplatys duboisi* with black-spot disease caused by a larval digenetic trematode (metacercaria) in the center of each black spot.

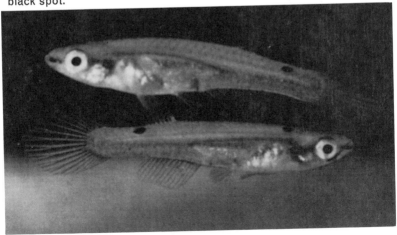

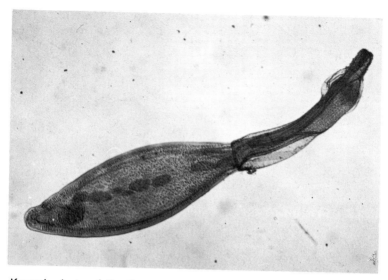

Knaack photo of the thorny-headed worm, *Echinorhynchus proteus*.

Q. brasiliensis	*Hoplias malabaricus,*	
	Hoplerythrinus	
	unitaeniatus	Brazil
Palliolisentis quinqueungulis	*Triportheus angulatus,*	
	T. paranensis	Brazil
P. ornatus	*T. paranensis*	Paraguay
Acanthosentis betwai	*Labeo gonius*	India
A. dattai	*Barbus ticto, B. stigma*	India
A. holospinus	*Barbus stigma*	India
A. maroccanus	*Barbus setivimensis*	Morocco
A. nigeriensis	*Labeo koubie*	Nigeria
A. sircari	*Rasbora elonga*	India
A. tilapiae	*Tilapia lidole*	Lake Malawi
	T. tanganicae	Tanganyika
Pallisentis basiri	*Trichogaster chuna*	India
P. colisai	*Colisa fasciatus*	India
P. nandai	*Nandus nandus*	India
P. ophiocephali	*Ophiocephalus* spp.	Asia
P. gaboes	*Ophiocephalus* spp.	Asia
P. nagpurensis	*Ophiocephalus* spp.	Asia
P. allahabadii	*Ophiocephalus* spp.	Asia
Raosentis podderi	*Mystus cavasius*	India
Echinorhynchus paranense	*Triportheus paranensis*	Brazil
E. salobrense	*Mylossoma paraguayensis*	Brazil

Filisoma indicum	Scatophagus argus	India, Celebes
F. hoogliensis	S. argus	India
F. rizalinum	S. argus	Philippines
F. scatophagusi	S. argus	India
Paracavisoma impudicum	Doras niger	Brazil
Tenuiproboscis misgurni	Misgurnus fossilis	Japan
Rhadinorhynchus horridum	Gnathonemus cyprinoides	Egypt
Paragorgorhynchus	Alestes dentax,	
albertianum	Schilbe mystus	Africa
Polyacanthorhynchus		
macrorhynchus	Arapaima gigas	Brazil
P. rhopalorhynchus	Arapaima gigas	Brazil
Atactorhynchus verecundus	Cyprinodon variegatus	Texas, Florida
Farzandia ophiocephali	Ophiocephalus striatus	Thailand
F. sp.	Ctenops vittatus	Thailand

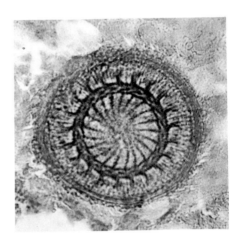

C. van Duijn, Jr. photomicrograph of the protozoan parasite *Cyclochaeta domerguei* from slime of a diseased fish; can cause skin discoloration.

Goldstein photo of discus with hole-in-the-head disease; though no worm-like extrusions are present, blotches indicate sites of eruption.

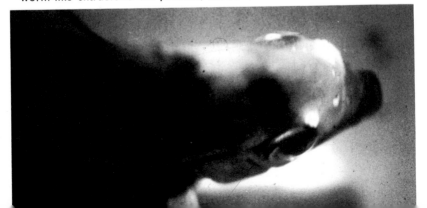

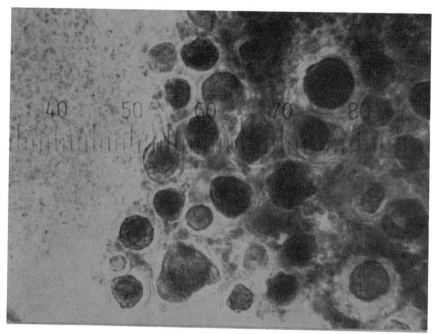

Liver of fish with advanced *Ichthyophonus* invasion. Photo by Helmert.

Zukal photo of *Xiphophorus* with fin rot attacking the tail fin.

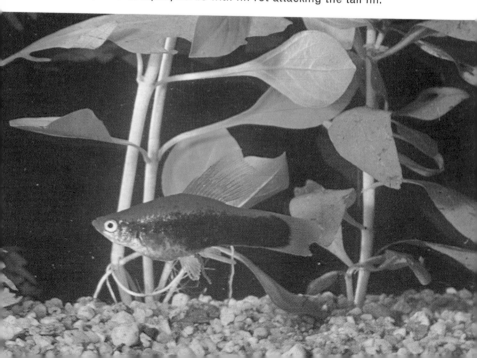

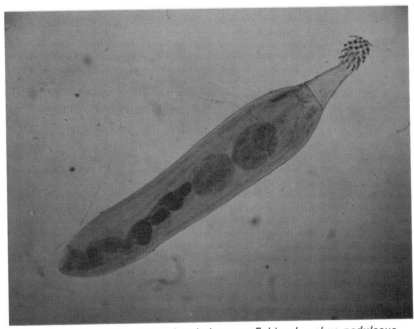

Knaack photo of the thorny-headed worm, *Echinorhynchus nodulosus.*

Xiphophorus maculatus with ichthyophthiriasis in an early stage. Photo by M. F. Roberts.

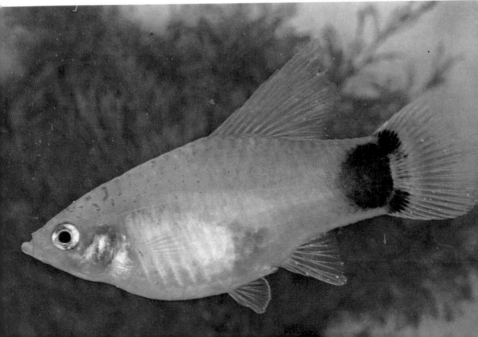

Below and opposite: Marcuse photos of a Hirudinean species of leech.

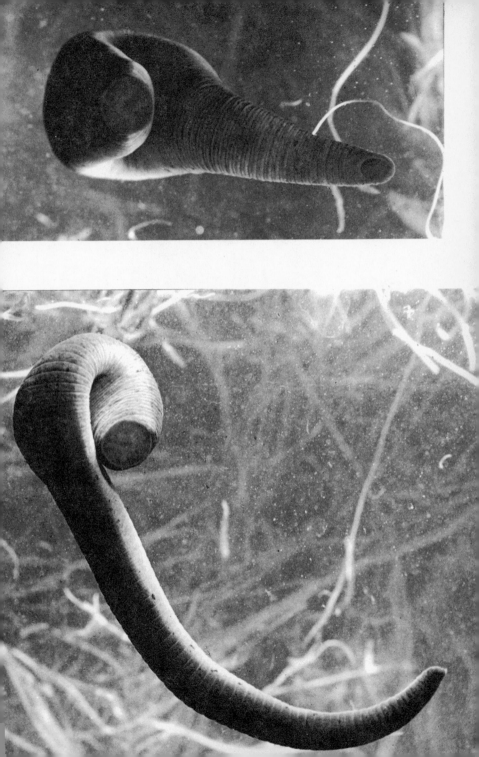

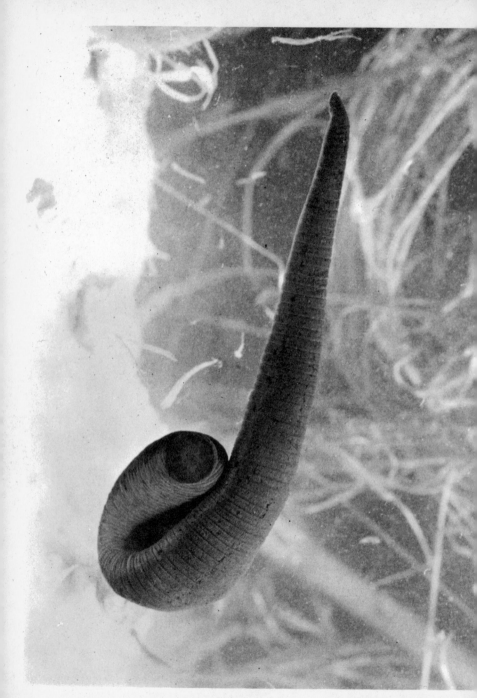

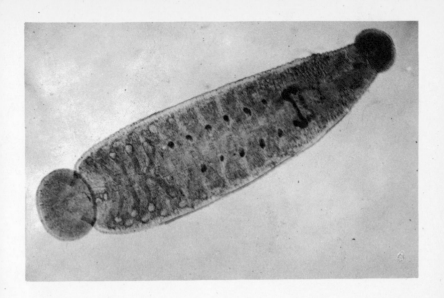

Leeches: Marcuse photo (opposite) of a Hirudinean species, and Knaack photos of *Hemiclepsis marginata* (above), and *Haemopsis sanguesuga*.

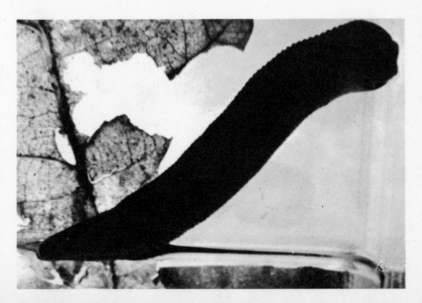

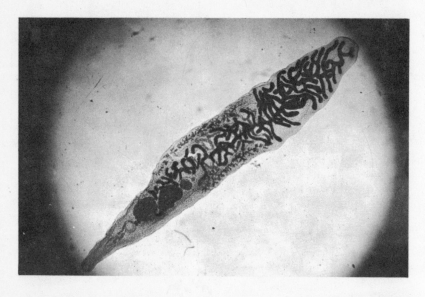

Parasitic worms: *Dicrocoelium lanceolatum* (above), and *Dicrocoelium cygnoides*. Knaack photos.

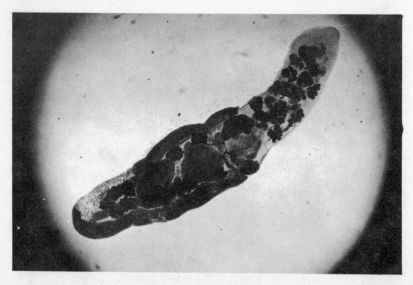

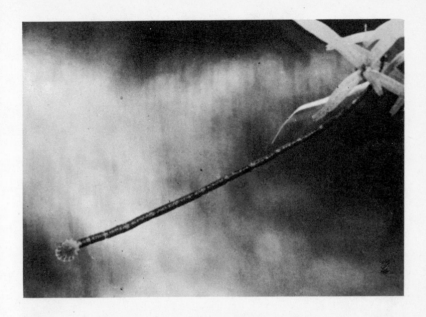

Helmert photo of the leech, *Piscicola geometra*, and (below) Schubert photo of eggs of the nematode, *Capillaria pterophylli.*

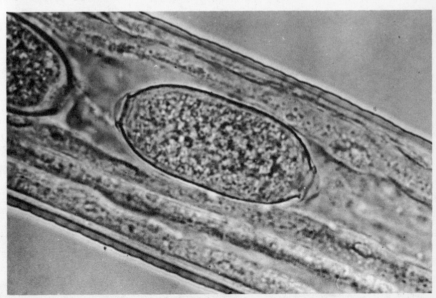

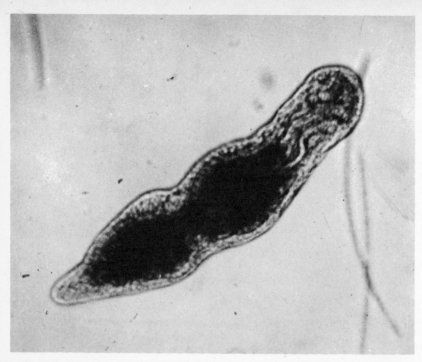

Turbellarian planarian photo by Helmert; (below) Schubert photo of
head of *Gyrodactylus* species.

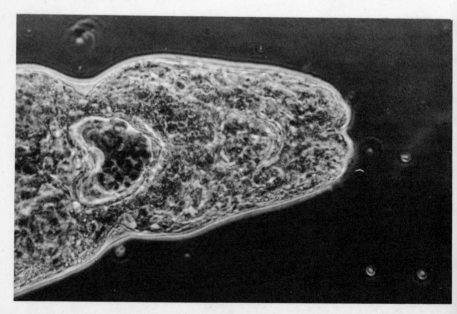

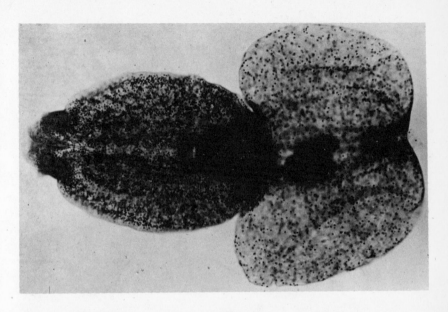

Schubert photos of larva of a fluke often found within imported discus-fishes, and (below) of attachment end of a gill fluke.

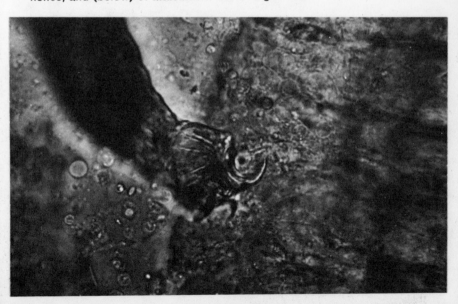

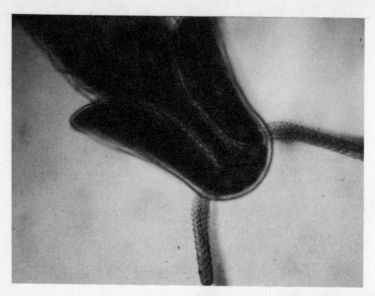

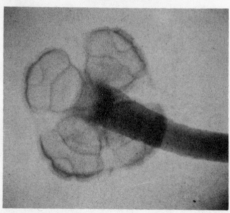

Scolex (head) of a trypanorhynch tapeworm from a cownosed ray (above), and that of a phyllobothriid tapeworm from a butterfly ray. Goldstein photos.

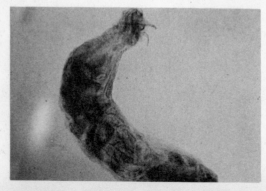

Goldstein photo of monogenetic trematode from the South American catfish, *Pseudoplatystoma fasciatum*.

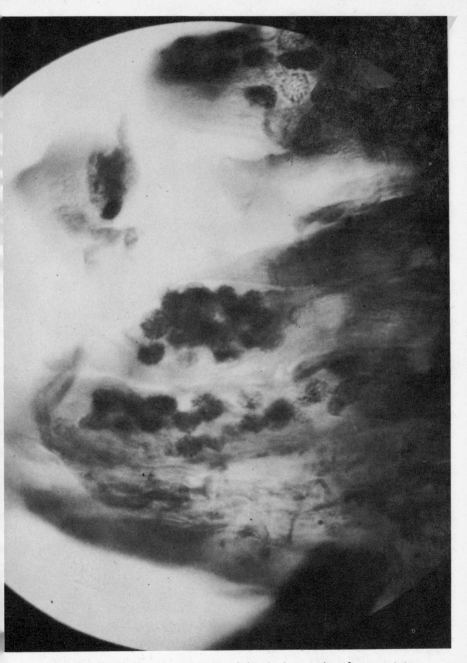

Plistophora hyphessobryconis in abdominal muscle of neon tetra.
Geisler photo.

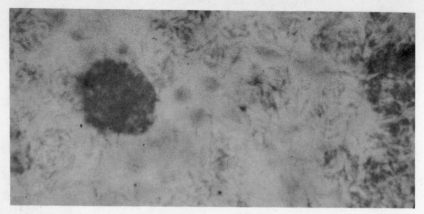

Mycobacterium piscium infection in *Rasbora heteromorpha*. Geisler photo.

21. PARASITIC CRUSTACEANS

The Phylum ARTHROPODA are jointed-legged animals with a hard outer skeleton. They have a number of affinities with segmented or annelid worms. The arthropods are divided into about six Classes, and one of these, the Class CRUSTACEA, contains many parasites of fishes.

A short breakdown of this Class will indicate how many animals you already know.

Subclass BRANCHIOPODA
    Order Anostraca   *Artemia* (brine shrimp)
Subclass OSTRACODA   *Cypris* (hardshell daphniae)
Subclass COPEPODA   *Cyclops*, anchor worm
Subclass BRANCHIURA   *Argulus* (fish louse)
Subclass CIRRIPEDIA   barnacles
Subclass MALACOSTRACA
    Order Peracarida
      Suborder Amphipoda   *Gammarus* (shrimp-imps)
      Suborder Isopoda   pill bugs
    Order Eucarida
      Suborder Decapoda   lobsters, shrimp, crabs

There are parasitic forms which attack fishes and other higher animals, and there are forms which parasitize other crustaceans. There are even males of a species which are said to parasitize the females, which in turn parasitize something else! The group is so large, however, and its biology so varied, that we are forced to limit our discussion to some generalizations and a few species of importance to most aquarists.

There are a number of larval stages before the final (adult) stage is reached. Some species are always parasitic, others only as adults, and others only as larvae. The remedies available to aquarists are very limited, and we will cover them in the proper places.

The Subclass BRANCHIURA contains the fish louse, *Argulus*, as well as other less well known genera: *Chonopeltis, Dolops, Huargulus, Dipteropeltis* and *Talaus* (the latter may be identical with *Dipteropeltis*). These are generally flattened animals, disc-shaped or arrowhead-shaped. There may be a pair of attachment discs (modified mouthparts of all things!), a distinct bifurcate tail of varying length, about four pairs of bristly legs, plus a couple of pairs of additional appendages up front. These parasites do not attach very firmly to the host fish, are not very host-specific, and may glide over the surface of many species, grazing on skin and mucus. Some species live in the mouths of fishes. Adults and larvae are parasitic and can swim to and from their hosts, except for *Chonopeltis* which cannot swim.

In light infections in the home aquarium, the fish can be removed in a net, and the parasites removed with a pair of tweezers or with the fingers. One can also slide a dull knife underneath them for removal. No intermediate host is required and a few parasites in an aquarium can multiply to epidemic proportions. The plants should be removed and the tank treated with fresh potassium permanganate solution. Commercial remedies are available, and the dose is not critical. The dye should turn the water a light maroon color. If the dye turns the water brown, it is too old to be effective and must be discarded. Tablets of permanganate can be purchased at your drug store. The average required dose is about one half grain per five gallons. As the dye may be taken up by peat moss, mulm and certain rocks, these should all be removed prior to treatment.

The Subclass MALACOSTRACA contains the isopods (and other animals), some of which are extraordinary parasites. Some typical free-living isopods you have seen are the pill bug, sow bug or armadillo bug, often seen in sidewalk cracks, under rocks or

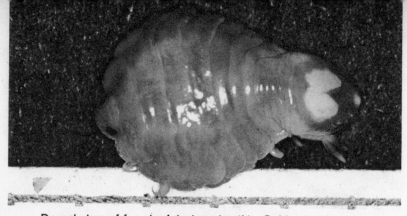

Dorsal view of female *Artystone trysibia*. Goldstein photo.

under decaying wood. These are little gray animals, with many segments, that roll up into a ball when frightened. Persons who have fished on coastal piers and rock jetties have seen myriads of segmented "bait-bugs" that clamber quickly out of every nook and cranny, and are forever getting into the cut bait.

The parasitic isopods are often gray or white, most of them marine, and many of them quite large. A few species have been found in or on fishes of aquarium interest. A parasitic isopod that occurs on the skin or in the mouth of a fish is easily removed with tweezers, but those that occur internally are often not seen until death, if then. There are no medications worth mentioning and infection is so rare as not to warrant it. Some isopods attack other crustaceans, often at specific sites in the body, and may even cause a parasitic castration as they destroy the host's gonads with their growth. There are many bizarre species, but most of the species attacking fishes bear a striking resemblance to a large pill bug, and are therefore easily recognized.

Badroulboudour and *Meinertia* occur in the mouths of fishes, *Lironeca* on the body surface and under the gill covers, and *Artystone* and *Ichthyoxenus* usually in the body cavity. These latter two genera probably invade the host skin as tiny larvae, and proceed to grow to large size inside. *Artystone trysibia* has been found in the body cavity of discus fish, and elsewhere, and occurs singly. It is South American. *Ichthyoxenus* occurs in Asian fishes, and a pair of them are always found in the same cyst. *Lironeca tanganyikae* occurs only on a single species of cichlid in Lake Tanganyika, whereas another species of the genus occurs on herringlike fishes in the same lake.

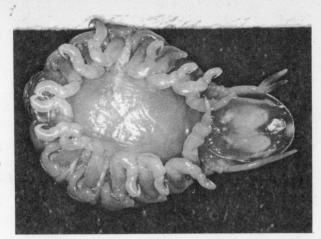

Artystone trysibia female from discusfish, ventral view. Photo by Goldstein.

The Subclass COPEPODA contains the copepods, a huge group with an enormous number of parasitic forms. Every aquarist has seen tiny *Cyclops* among his live *Daphnia* or in a tank being given infusoria for fry.

There are only a small number of genera of interest to us as aquarists, but some of these genera contain a goodly number of species.

Every pondfish keeper, or aquarist who has seen large goldfish, has also seen cases of *anchor worm*. This is the name given to various species of the genus *Lernaea* (family Lernaeidae). Anchor worms are bizarre cases of excessive modification associated with parasitism. One of the early larval stages looks like any other copepod. It seeks out a species of fish and attaches to the fish's

A *Lernaea* species dissected out of a native pickerel. Goldstein photo.

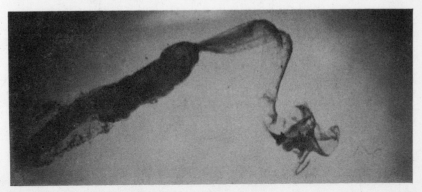

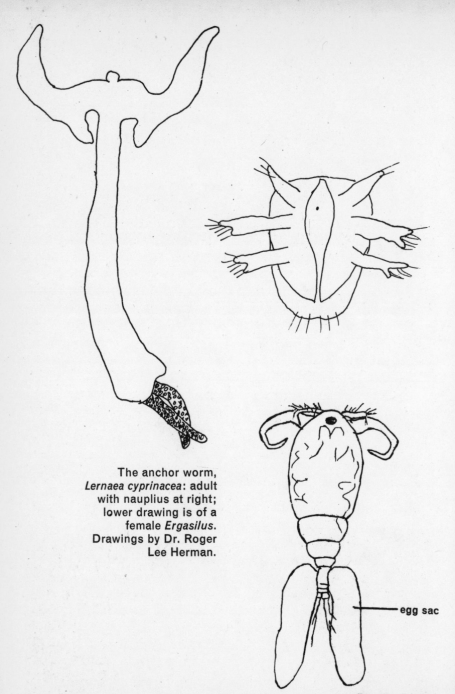

The anchor worm, *Lernaea cyprinacea*: adult with nauplius at right; lower drawing is of a female *Ergasilus*. Drawings by Dr. Roger Lee Herman.

egg sac

Ergasilus female

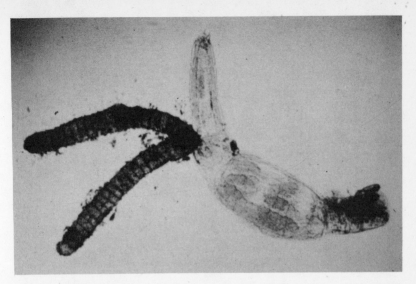

Lamproglena monodi from a *Tilapia macrochir* of Togo; the parasite is specific for the gills of African fishes, especially cichlids. Goldstein photo.

gills. Here it is nourished by the fluids it draws from this host, and the parasite grows and modifies. Finally, it releases its hold and becomes free-swimming, mature and in search of a mate. After mating has occurred in the open waters only the female resumes the parasitic mode of life. She seeks out a fish (usually of a different species than before) and buries her head in its flesh. Now the great modification comes about. The head begins to modify, perhaps with a few horns, or sometimes with excessive branching like the roots of a tree. How these rhizoidal (branching) extensions of the head receive nourishment is not clear, because the whole thing becomes encased in a host-produced capsule of connective tissue, in an immune response which (in vain) tries to isolate this foreign tissue from the tissues of the host. This connective tissue seems impervious to fluids from the host, but apparently the parasite knows something we don't know. At the same time, one of the body segments of the parasite, on the outside of the host, begins to greatly elongate. Finally, this segment is so long as to resemble a stick or a worm. It juts from the side of the fish, while the head or "anchor" is imbedded (often deeply) within the fish. In some species the head, when cut out, resembles a marine anchor.

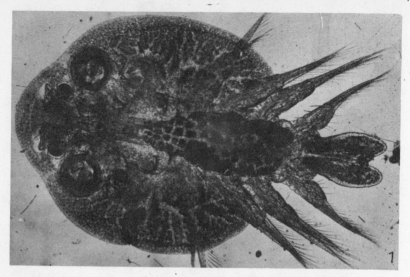

Knaack photo of ventral view of freshwater fish louse, *Argulus*.

What can you do to treat anchor worm? Practically nothing. Once the fish is seen to have the adult female parasite jutting from its side, all you can do is try to pull it out with a tweezers (if not very deep), or cut the elongate segment close to the surface of the fish. The wound should then be swabbed with mercurochrome (home preparations work fine), and the aquarist can only hope that a gangrenous infection doesn't follow. If the parasite is imbedded close to the eye or brain, or if there are only a very few of them, it is best to leave the fish untreated. Surgery should only be performed if the infection is massive and the fish is expected to die anyway, or if the fish is cheap and the parasite is in a relatively muscular and safe area.

In pond fish culture (or outdoor goldfish or *Tilapia* pools), one may treat the water with Chemagro Corporation's Dylox®, an organic insecticide. Some other insecticides contain the same active ingredient, 0,0-dimethyl, 2,2,2-trichloro-1-hydroxyethyl phosphonate. This drug is relatively non-toxic to mammals, compared with other organophosphate insecticides. It is used in cold water situations, because it rapidly breaks down at warm

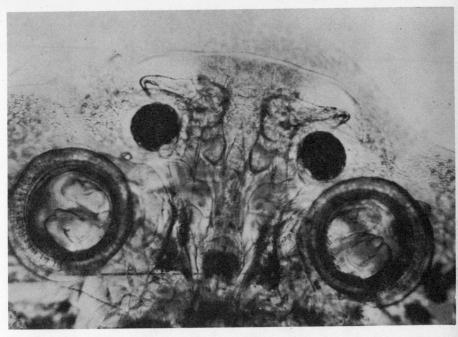

Detail of head of *Argulus*, with eyes and sucking discs prominently shown. Knaack photo.

Goldstein photo below is of a fish louse from the skin of a marine fish.

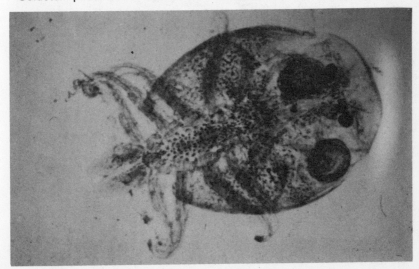

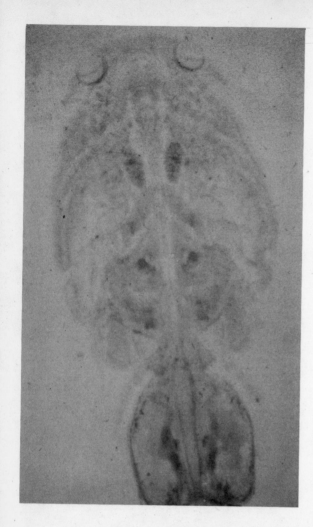

Caligus, a crustacean parasite of fishes. Goldstein photo.

temperatures. Since the anchor worm has a life cycle of about three weeks, it is necessary to continue treatment for prolonged periods. The dosage may vary from 0.25 to 0.5 p.p.m. At high drug concentrations, especially over a long period of time, the fishes may develop curvature of the spine. Thus, the drug should be measured out carefully. It hits all stages of the parasites, and appears to be an excellent control in ponds.

In aquaria, the life cycle doesn't generally occur, and only adult parasites are found. There is no information at present on the use of the drug in warm water aquaria.

The Lernaeidae of African fishes have received much attention in recent years. Some of the genera found there are *Lernaea*, *Afrolernaea*, *Lamproglena* and *Lamproglenoides*. In the United States we find *Lernaea*, *Achtheres*, and *Salmincola*.

Other parasitic copepods are *Caligus* (in the gill chambers of marine fishes) and *Ergasilus* (in the gill cavity of freshwater and marine fishes). *Ergasilus* species are very small parasites, difficult to detect unless you are examining the gills with a hand lens. The genus is easily identified by the large pair of claspers at the front end of the parasite. Only the female is parasitic, and so every parasite you see may be carrying a pair of elongate egg sacs. (These egg sacs are often seen as well in *Lernaea*). These copepods are generally not very host-specific in nature, and are even less so in aquaria. *Ergasilus* does not require an intermediate host; thus one can get epidemics in aquaria. Treatment is with potassium permanganate, as for *Argulus*.

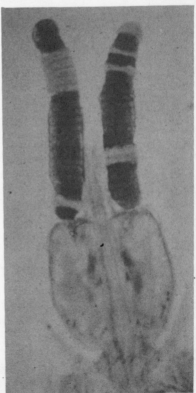

Egg sacs on a female *Caligus*. Photo by Goldstein.

22. PARASITIC CRUSTACEANS FROM FISHES OF AQUARIUM INTEREST

Parasite	Host	Locality
Branchiura		
Argulus africanus	*Heterobranchus, Clarias, Lates, Bagrus, Protopterus, Mormyrus, Mormyrops, Eutropius, Barbus, Schilbe, Labeo, Tilapia*	Africa
A. ambloplites	*Ophiocephalus, Clarias, Hydrocyon*	Africa
A. americanus	*Amia calva*	North America
A. angusticeps	Free in Lake Tanganyika	Africa
A. brachypeltis	*Hydrocyon lineatus* (N. Rhodesia)	Africa
A. carteri	*Hoplias malabaricus* (Brazil, Paraguay)	South America
A. cenotae	*Rhamdia guatemalensis* (Yucatan)	Central America
A. chinensis	*Ophiocephalus argus,. Leiocassis* sp.	China
A. chromidis	*Chromis, Rhamdia* (Nicaragua, Yucatan)	Central America
A. capensis	Capetown, South Africa (hosts?)	Africa
A. cubensis	*Cichlasoma tetracanthus* (Cuba)	Carribean
A. exiguus	*Haplocheilus tanganicus, Simochromis diagramma* (Lake Tanganyika)	Africa
A. flavescens	*Amia calva, Floridichthys carpio*	North America
A. incisus	*Auchenoglanis occidentalis*	Africa
A. indicus	*Trichopterus pectoralis* (Thailand)	Asia
A. juparanensis	*Astyanax bimaculatus*	Brazil
A. monodi	*Hydrocyon lineatus* (Lake Bangweulu)	Africa
A. reticulatus	*Hydrocyon goliath* (Congo)	Africa
A. rhipidiophorus	*Hydrocyon, Clarias* (Lakes, Albert and Rudolph)	Africa
A. schoutedeni	*Distichodus fasciolatus, Hydrocyon,* (*Mormyrus, Marcusenius* doubtfully)	Africa
A. siamensis	*Ophiocephalus, Labeo rohita, Ambassis ranga*	India
A. striatus	*Clarias, Auchenoglanis*	Africa
A. vierai	*Cnesterodon decemmaculatus* (Uruguay)	South America
A. violaceus	*Rhamdia, Plecostomus, Hoplias, Loricaria, Pimelodus*	South America

A. wilsoni	*Hydrocyon goliath*	Africa
Dolops ranarum	*Schilbe, Clarias, Eutropius,*	
	Heterobranchus, Bagrus	Africa
D. discoidalis	*Hoplias, Phractocephalus*	South America
D. geayi	*Hoplias malabaricus, Aequidens*	
	pulcher, Crenicichla geayi	South America
Huargulus chinensis	*Ophiocephalus argus*	China
Dipteropeltis hirundo	*Curimatus* sp. (Argentina)	South America
Chonopeltis inermis	*Clarias mossambicus*	Africa
C. brevis	*Cyprinidae (Barbus, Labeo)*	Africa
C. congicus	*Gnathonemus monteiri*	Africa
C. flaccifrons	*Marcusenius* spp. (Mormyridae)	Africa
C. meridionalis	*Labeo rosae* and other cyprinids	Africa
C. schoutedeni	Mormyridae	Africa
Copepoda		
Ergasilus sarsi	*Tylochromis mylodon* (cichlid),	
	Gnathonemus macrolepidotus,	
	Synodontis nigromaculatus,	
	Clarias mellandi	Africa
E. kandti	*Pelmatochromis congicus*	Africa
E. megacheir	*Pelmatochromis congicus*	Africa
E. cunningtoni	*Mormyrops nigricans, Gnatho-*	
	nemus moorei, G. greshoffi,	
	Marcusenius isidori, Eutropius	
	laticeps, Distichodus	
	atroventralis, Tylochromis	
	lateralis, Pelmatochromis	
	congicus	Africa
Lernaea barnimiana	*Tilapia melanopleura, Labeo*	
	altivelis	Africa
L. palati	*Haplochromis chrysonotus,*	
	H. nkatae (Lake Malawi)	Africa
L. tilapiae	*Tilapia* spp.	Africa
L. bagri	*Bagrus* spp.	Africa
L. haplocephala	*Polypterus* spp.	Africa
L. hardingi	*Chrysichthys mabusi, Synodontis*	
	nigromaculatus, Sargochromis	
	mellandi (and other cichlids)	Africa
Opistholernaea		
laterobrachialis	*Tilapia macrochir*	Africa
O. longa	*Lates* spp.	Africa
Lamproglenoides		
vermiformis	*Labeo cylindricus*	Africa
Afrolernaea		
longicollis	Mormyridae	Africa
A. nigeriensis	Mormyridae	Africa

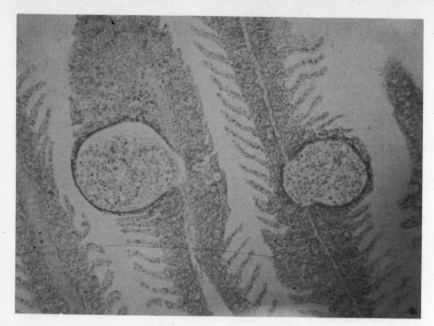

Myxosoma (above), and a rat-tailed maggot, syrphid larva of a fly which lays its eggs in waters containing rotted vegetation. It survives in the intestines of persons who have ingested it while eating watercress and causes digestive upset, nervous symptoms, and foul breath; it can probably survive in the gut of fishes as well. Goldstein photos.

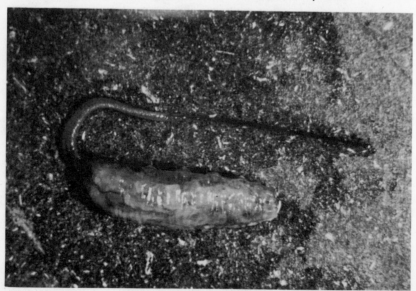

Parasite	Host	Locality
Lamproglena wilsoni	*Clarotes* (Bagridae)	Africa
L. elongata	Characidae, Citharinidae	Africa
L. hemprichii	Characidae	Africa
L. monodi	Cichlidae	Africa
L. clarii	Clariidae	Africa
L. barbicola	*Barbus* spp.	Africa
L. intercedens	Citharinidae	Africa
L. cleopatra	*Lates* spp.	Africa
L. werneri	*Bagrus* spp.	Africa
L. angusta	*Malapterurus* spp.	Africa
Isopoda		
Lironeca expansus	*Eugnathichthys eetveldii* (Congo)	Africa
L. tanganyikae	*Simochromis diagramma* (Lake Tanganyika)	Africa
Artystone trysibia	*Symphysodon, Crenicichla, Geophagus, Corydoras, Anostomus,* tetra	South America
Ichthyoxenus jellinghausii	*Nemacheilus*	Asia
I. montanus	*Barbus sophores* (Himalayas)	Asia
I. japonicus	several species	Asia
Badroulboudour sp.	Loricariidae	Ecuador

Cymothoid parasite (crustacean) from a fish. Goldstein photo.

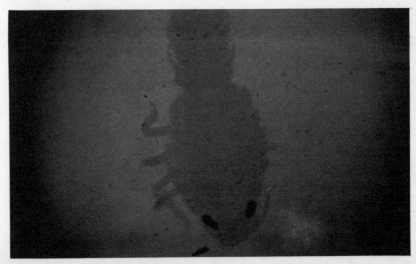

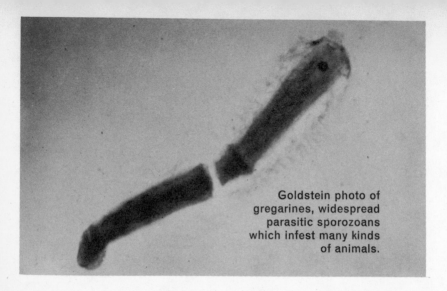

Goldstein photo of gregarines, widespread parasitic sporozoans which infest many kinds of animals.

Geisler photo of a platy-swordtail cross with tumor in the tail, showing pigmentation and accumulation of giant cells.

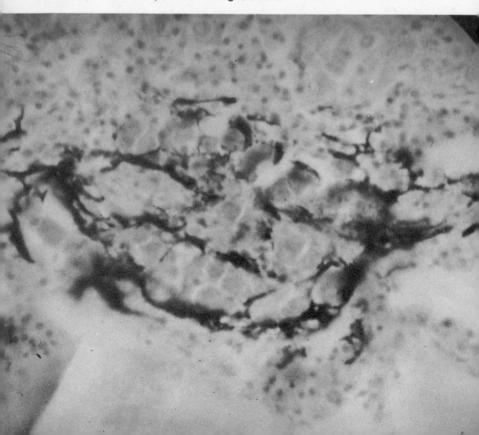

BIBLIOGRAPHY

Ajmal, M., and Hobbs, B. C. 1967. Columnaris disease in roach and perch from English waters. Species of *Corynebacterium* and *Pasteurella* isolated from diseased salmon, trout and rudd. **Nature 215:** 141–143.

Anderson, J. I. W., and Conroy, D. A. 1969. The pathogenic myxobacteria with special reference to fish diseases. **J. App. Bact. 32:** 30–39.

Anderson, P. D., and Battle, H. I. 1967. Effects of chloramphenicol on the development of the zebrafish, *Brachydanio rerio*. **Canad. J. Zool. 45:** 191–204.

Becker, C. D., and Katz, M. 1965. *Babesiosoma tetragonis* n.sp. (Sporozoa: Dactlyosomidae) from a California teleost. **J. Protozool. 12:** 189–193.

Bullock, G. L. 1961. A schematic outline for the presumptive identification of bacterial diseases of fish. **Prog. Fish Cult. 23:** 147–151.

—— 1965. Simple enrichment of commercial media for growth of *Hemophilus piscium*. **Prog. Fish Cult. 27:** 163–164.

——, Snieszko, S. F., and Dunbar, C. E. 1965. Characteristics and identification of oxidative pseudomonads isolated from diseased fish. **J. Gen. Microbiol. 38:** 1–7.

Bullock, W. 1957. The acanthocephalan parasites of fishes of the Texas coast. **Bull. Inst. Mar. Sci. 4:** 278–283.

—— 1960. Some acanthocephalan parasites of Florida fishes. **Bull. Mar. Sci. Gulf and Carib. 10:** 481–484.

Dawes, B. *The Trematoda, with special reference to British and other European forms,* Cambridge University Press, 1956, 644p.

Dias, F. F., Agate, A. D., Bhat, J. V., Pillai, S. C., and Aswathanarayana, N.V. 1965. *Aeromonas punctata* in *Puntius* species. **Curr. Sci. 34:** 81–82.

Dunbar, C. E., and Wolf, K. 1966. The cytological course of experimental lymphocystis in the bluegill. **J. Infect. Dis. 116:** 466–472.

Erickson, J. D. 1965. Report on the problem of *Ichthyosporidium* in rainbow trout. **Prog. Fish Cult. 27:** 179–183.

Fernando, C. H., and Furtado, J. I. 1963a. Some studies on helminth parasites of freshwater fishes. **Proc. First Reg. Sympos. Sci. Knowledge Trop. Parasites,** U. Singapore, 5–9 Nov., 1962, 293–302.

—— —— 1963b. A study of some helminth parasites of freshwater fishes in Ceylon. **Z.f. Parasit. 23:** 141–163.

—— —— 1963c. Helminth parasites of some Malayan fresh-water fishes. **Bull. Nat. Mus., Singapore, 32:** 45–71.

Fryer, G. 1964. Further studies on the parasitic crustacea of African freshwater fishes. **Proc. Zool. Soc. London 143:** 79–102.

—— 1968. A new parasitic isopod of the family Cymothoidae from clupeid fishes of Lake Tanganyika—a further Lake Tanganyika enigma. **J. Zool. London 156:** 35–43.

—— 1968b. The parasitic crustacea of African freshwater fishes; their biology and distribution. **J. Zool. London 156:** 45–95.

Goldstein, R. J. 1965. The sheepshead minnow heart fluke. **J. Amer. Killifish Assoc. 2:** 11–12.

Gopalakrishnan, V. 1964. Recent developments in the prevention and control of parasites of fishes cultured in Indian waters. **Proc. Zool. Soc. Calcutta 17:** 95–100.

Griffin, P. J., and Snieszko, S. F. 1951. A unique bacterium pathogenic for warm-blooded and cold-blooded animals. **Fishery Bull. Fish Wildlife Serv. 52:** 187–190.

Hoffman, G. L. 1963. Parasites of freshwater fish. 1. Fungi (*Saprolegnia* and relatives) of fish and fish eggs. **U.S.D.I., F.W.S. Fishery leaflet 564:** 1–6.

—— 1965. *Eimeria aurati* n. sp. (Protozoa: Eimeriidae) from goldfish (*Carassius auratus*) in North America. **J. Protozool. 12:** 273–275.

—— *Parasites of North American Freshwater Fishes,* Univ. California Press, Berkeley and Los Angeles, 1967, 486 p.

——, Dunbar, C. E., and Bradford, A. 1962. Whirling disease of trouts caused by *Myxosoma cerebralis* in the United States. **U.S.D.I., F.W.S., Spec. Sci. rep. 427:** 1–15.

——, Putz, R. E., and Dunbar, C. E. 1965. Studies on *Myxosoma cartilaginis* n. sp. (Protozoa: Myxosporidea) of centrarchid fish and a synopsis of the *Myxosoma* of North American freshwater fishes. **J. Protozool. 12:** 319–332.

Kluge, J. P. 1965. A tranulomatous disease of fish produced by flavobacteria. **Path. Vet. 2:** 545–552.

Kohn, A., and Paperna, I. 1964. Monogenetic trematodes from aquarium fishes. **Rev. Brasil. Biol. 24:** 145–149.

Lanzing, W. J. R. 1965. Observations on malachite green in relation to its application to fish diseases. **Hydrobiol. 25:** 426–440.

Lawler, A. R. 1967. *Oodinium cyprinodontum* n. sp., a parasitic dinoflagellate on gills of Cyprinodontidae of Virginia. **Chesapeake Sci. 8:** 67–68.

—— 1968a. New host record for the parasitic dinoflagellate *Oodinium cyprinodontum* Lawler, 1967. **Chesapeake Sci. 9:** 263.

—— 1968b. Occurrence of the parasitic dinoflagellate *Oodinium cyprinodontum* Lawler, 1967 in North Carolina. **Virginia J. Sci. 19:** 240.

Lom, J., and Corliss, J. O. 1967. Ultrastructural observations on the development of the microsporidian protozoon *Plistophora hyphessobryconis* Schaperclaus. **J. Protozool. 14:** 141–152.

——, and Hoffman, G. L. 1964. Geographic distribution of some species of trichodinids (Ciliata: Peritricha) parasitic on fishes. **J. Parasit. 50:** 30–35.

Mackiewicz, J. S., and Beverley-Burton, M. 1967. *Monobothrioides woodlandi* sp. nov. (Cestoidea: Caryophyllidea) from *Clarias mellandi* Boulenger (Cypriniformes: Clariidae) in Zambia, Africa. **Proc. Helm. Soc. Washington 34:** 125–128.

Meyer, F. P. 1966. A new control for the anchor parasite, *Lernaea cyprinacea*. **Prog. Fish Cult. 28:** 33–39.

Midlige, F. H., Jr., and Malsberger, R. G. 1968. In vitro morphology and maturation of lymphocystis virus. **J. Virol. 2:** 830–835.

Mizelle, J. D., Kritsky, D. C., and Crane, J. W. 1968. Studies on monogenetic trematodes. XXXVIII. Ancyrocephalinae from South America with the proposal of *Jainus* gen. n. **Amer. Midland Natur. 80:** 186–198.

——, and Price, C. E. 1965. Studies on monogenetic trematodes. XXVIII. Gill parasites of the piranha with proposal of *Anacanthorus* gen. n. **J. Parasit. 51:** 30–36.

Paperna, I. 1960. Studies on monogenetic trematodes in Israel. 2. Monogenetic trematodes of cichlids. **Bamidgeh 12:** 20–33.

—— 1963. *Enterogyrus cichlidarum* n. gen., n. sp., a monogenetic trematode parasitic in the intestine of a fish. **Bull. Res. Conc. Israel 11B:** 183–187.

—— 1965. Monogenetic trematodes collected from fresh water fish in southern Ghana. **Bamidgeh 17:** 107–111.

—— 1968a. Monogenetic trematodes collected from fresh water fish in Ghana. Second Report. **Bamidgeh 20:** 88–100.

—— 1968b. *Onchobdella* n. gen. New genus of monogenetic trematodes (Dactylogyridae, Bychowski 1933) from cichlid fish from West Africa. **Proc. Helm. Soc. Washington 35:** 200–206.

—— 1968c. Ectoparasitic infections on fish of Volta Lake, Ghana. **Bull. Wildlife Dis. Assoc. 4:** 135–137.

——, and Thurston, J. P. 1969 Monogenetic trematodes (Dactylogyridae) from fish in Uganda. **Rev. Zool. Bot. Afr. 78:** 284–294.

Pearse, A. S. 1933. Parasites of Siamese fishes and crustaceans. **J. Siam Soc., Nat. Hist. Suppl. 9:** 179–191.

Pfeiffer, W. 1962. The fright reaction of fish. **Biol. Rev. 37:** 495–511.

Powles, P. M., Garnett, D. G., Ruggieri, G. D., and Nigrelli, R. F. 1968. *Ichthyophonus* infection in yellowtail flounder (*Limanda ferruginea*) off Nova Scotia. **J. Fish. Res. Bd. Can. 25:** 597–598.

Premvati, G. 1969. Studies on *Haplobothrium bistrobilae* sp. nov. (Cestoda: Pseudophyllidea) from *Amia calva* L. **Proc. Helm. Soc. Washington 36:** 55–60.

Price, C. E. 1966. *Urocleidus cavanaughi*, a new monogenetic trematode from the gills of the keyhole cichlid, *Aequidens maroni* (Steindachner). **Bull. Ga. Acad. Sci. 24:** 117–120.

—— 1967a. The freshwater monogenetic trematodes of Africa. **Rev. Zool. Bot. Afr. 76:** 375–391.

—— 1967b. The freshwater monogenetic trematodes of South America. **Riv. di Parassit. 28:** 87–95.

——, and Arai, H. P. 1967. A proposed system of anatomy for freshwater monogenea. **Can. J. Zool. 45:** 1283–1285.

——, and Bussing, W. A. 1967. Monogenean parasites of Costa Rican fishes. Part 1. Descriptions of two new species of *Cleidodiscus* Mueller, 1934. **Riv. di Parassit. 28:** 81–86.

—— —— 1968. Monogenean parasites of Costa Rican fishes. II. Proposal of *Palombitrema heteroancistrium* n. gen., n. sp. **Proc. Helm. Soc. Washington 35:** 54–57.

——, and Schlueter, E. A. 1968. Two new monogenetic trematodes from South America. **J. Tenn. Acad. Sci. for 1968:** 23–25.

Pritchard, H. N., and Malsberger, R. G. 1968. A cytochemical study of lymphocystis tumor cells in vivo. **J. Exp. Zool. 169:** 371–380.

Putz, R. E. 1964. Parasites of freshwater fish. II. Protozoa. 1. Microsporidea of fish. **U.S.D.I., F.W.S., Fish. leaflet 571:** 1–4.

——, Hoffman, G. L., and Dunbar, C. E. Two new species of *Plistophora* (Microsporidea) from North American fish with a synopsis of microsporidea of freshwater and euryhaline fishes. **J. Protozool. 12:** 228–236.

Ramadevi, P., and Hanumantha Rao, K. 1966. Plerocercoid of *Senga* sp. (Pseudophyllidea: Ptychobothriidae) from the freshwater fish *Panchax panchax* (Ham. and Buch.). **Curr. Sci. 35:** 626–627.

Reichenbach-Klinke, H. H. 1968. Bemerkungen zu der arbeit von Ch. Meske, J. Meyer-Rohn und P. Schmidt *Ichthyophthirius multifilis* als möglicher parasit des menschen., **Z. Tropeenmed. Parasit. 18,** 330–333. **Z.f. Tropenmed. und Parasit. 19:** 342–343.

Schubert, G. 1967. *Henneguya pinnae* n. sp. aus den flossen von *Ctenopoma kingsleyae* Günther (Osteoichthyes, Anabantidae). **Z.f. Parasit. 29:** 304–309.

—— 1968. Electronenmikroskopische untersuchungen zur sporenentwicklung von *Henneguya pinnae* Schubert (Sporozoa, Myxosporidea, Myxobolidae). **Z.f. Parasit. 30:** 57–77.

Skidmore, J. F. 1964. Toxicity of zinc compounds to aquatic animals, with special reference to fish. **Quart. Rev. Biol. 39:** 227–248.

Snieszko, S. F., *editor*. 1964. *Symposium on Fish Microbiology*. **Dev. Industr. Microbiol. 5:** 97–148, A.I.B.S., Washington, D.C.

——, and Bullock, G. L. 1965. Freshwater fish diseases caused by bacteria belonging to the genera *Aeromonas* and *Pseudomonas*. **U.S.D.I., F.W.S., fishery leaflet 459:** 1–4.

Sogandares-Bernal, F., and Lumsden, R. D. 1964. The heterophyid trematode *Ascocotyle* (*A.*) *leighi* Burton, 1956, from the hearts of certain Poeciliid and Cyprinodont fishes. **Z.f. Parasit. 24:** 3–12.

Sprague, V. 1966. *Ichthyosporidium* sp. Schwartz, 1963, parasite of the fish *Leiostomus xanthurus*, is a microsporidian. **J. Protozool. 13:** 356–358.

——, and Vernick, S. H. 1968. Observations on the spores of *Pleistophora gigantea* (Thelohan, 1895) Swellengrebel, 1911, a microsporidian parasite of the fish *Crenilabrus melops*. **J. Protozool. 15:** 662–665.

Turnbull, E. R. 1956. *Gyrodactylus bullatarudis* n. sp. from *Lebistes reticulatus* Peters with a study of its life cycle. **Canad. J. Zool. 34:** 583–594.

Van Duijn, C., Jr. *Diseases of Fishes,* Chas. Thomas, Publ., Springfield, Illinois, U.S.A., 1967, second ed., 309 p.

Walker, R., and Weissenberg, R. 1965. Conformity of light and electron microscopic studies on virus particle distribution in lymphocystis tumor cells of fish. **Ann. N.Y. Acad. Sci. 126:** 375–385.

Wardle, R. A., and McLeod, J. A. *The Zoology of Tapeworms,* Oxford Univ. Press, London, 1952, 780 p.

Weissenberg, R. 1965a. Fifty years of research on the lymphocystis virus disease of fishes. **Ann. N.Y. Acad. Sci. 126:** 362–374.

—— 1965b. Morphological studies on lymphocystis tumor cells of a cichlid from Guatemala, *Cichlasoma synspilum* Hubbs. **Ann. N.Y. Acad. Sci. 126:** 396–413.

—— 1968. Intracellular development of the microsporidian *Glugea anomala* Moniez in hypertrophying migratory cells of the fish *Gasterosteus aculeatus* L., an example of the formation of "Xenoma" tumors. **J. Protozool. 15:** 44–57.

Wellborn, T. L., Jr. 1967. *Trichodina* (Ciliata: Urceolariidae) of freshwater fishes of the southeastern United States. **J. Protozool. 14:** 399–412.

Wolf, K., Gravell, M., and Malsberger, R. G. 1966. Lymphocystis virus: isolation and propagation in Centrarchid fish cell lines. **Science 151:** 1004–1005.

——, and Snieszko, S. F. 1964. Uses of antibiotics and other antimicrobials in therapy of diseases of fishes. **Antimicrobial Agents and Chemotherapy—1963:** 597–603.

Yamaguti, S. *Systema Helminthum, vol. 1, The digenetic trematodes of vertebrates,* Intersc. Publ., 1958, 1575 p.

—— *Systema Helminthum, vol. 2, The cestodes of vertebrates,* Intersc. Publ., 1959, 860 p.

—— *Systema Helminthum, vol. 4, Monogenea and Aspidocotylea,* Intersc. Publ., 1963, 699 p.

—— *Systema Helminthum, vol. 5, Acanthocephala,* Intersc. Publ., 1963, 423 p.

—— *Parasitic copepoda and branchiura of fishes,* Intersc. Publ., 1963, 1104 p.

Zwillenberg, L. O., and Wolf, K. 1968. Ultrastructure of lymphocystis virus. **J. Virol. 2:** 393–399.